Fix Your Body Chemistry

Also by Ya-Ling J. Liou D.C.

Put Out the Fire: "It Never Used to Hurt When I...?!"
(The Everyday Pain Guide, Volume 1)

Fix the Fire Damage: Your go-to guide when pain first strikes
(The Everyday Pain Guide, Volume 2)

Fix Your Body Mechanics: Companion Manual & Journal
(The Everyday Pain Guide Workbooks #1)

Fix Your Body Chemistry: Companion Manual & Journal
(The Everyday Pain Guide Workbooks #2)

Fix Your Stress Biology: Companion Manual & Journal
(The Everyday Pain Guide Workbooks #3)

The Everyday Pain Guide
WORKBOOKS

VOL.2
FIX THE
FIRE DAMAGE!

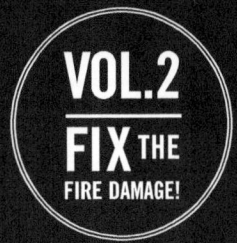

Fix Your Body Chemistry

COMPANION MANUAL & JOURNAL

YA-LING J. LIOU, D.C.

Artwork by SANDY JOHNSON

RETURN TO HEALTH PRESS

SEATTLE, WA

FIX YOUR BODY CHEMISTRY COMPANION MANUAL & JOURNAL
(THE EVERYDAY PAIN GUIDE WORKBOOKS #2)
© 2025 Ya-Ling J. Liou, D.C.
All rights reserved.

Published by Return to Health Press, Seattle, WA
Ya-Ling J. Liou, D.C., is a chiropractic physician in Seattle, WA
www.returntohealthpress.com

Notice
The information, techniques and suggestions contained in this book are not intended as a substitute for individual medical care. All matters regarding your health require medical supervision. Consult your health care professional before performing any exercise or taking any dietary supplement referenced in this book. Neither the author, nor the publisher, contributors or editors shall be liable or responsible for any loss, damage or risk arising, directly or indirectly, from the use and application of any of the contents of this book.

Cover Design by VMC Art & Design, LLC
Interior Design by VMC Art & Design, LLC
Image & Diagram Credits: 1983 Wong-Baker FACES Foundation. www.wongbakerfaces.org
Illustrations by Sandy Johnson

First Edition, 2025
Printed in the United States of America

ISBN: 978-0-9913094-5-0

CONTENTS

Author's Note

For best results, make sure to seek care as soon as possible and/or in conjunction with these strategies. Always check with a healthcare provider first.

SURPRISE PAIN?

Neck/Shoulder

Mid Back/Torso/Ribs

Neck

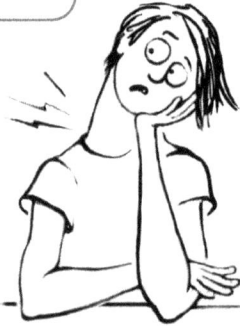

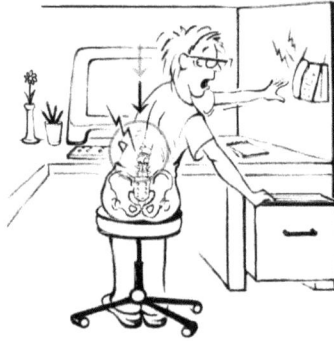

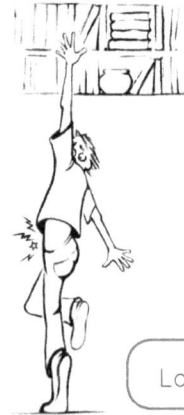

Low Back

Shoulder/Upper Back

Hip/Buttock/Thigh

Low Back/Hip

☑ BODY MECHANICS ACTION PLANS

➡ **BODY CHEMISTRY ACTION PLAN**

☑ STRESS BIOLOGY ACTION PLAN

1. RELEASE

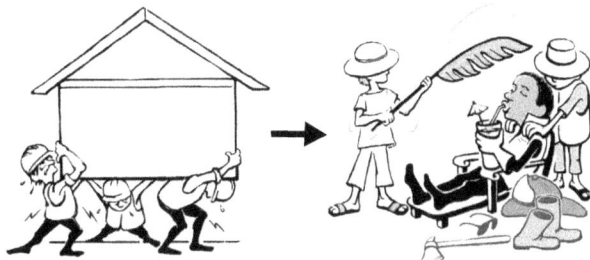

- *Mechanical Strain*
- **Body Chemistry Garbage**
- *Emotional Stress Triggers*

2. RETRAIN

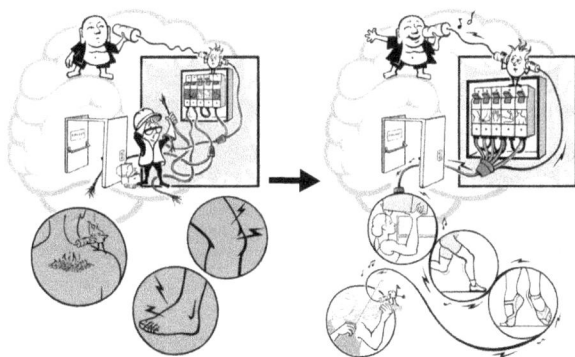

- *Body-Brain Connection*
- **Garbage Journeys**
- *Nervous System*

3. REINFORCE

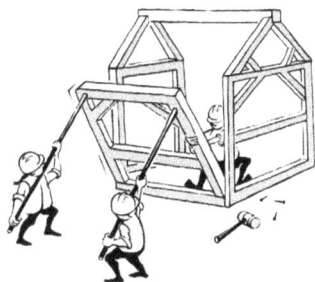

- *Mechanical Structure*
- **Garbage Elimination**
- *Low-Stress Biology*

IS IT TIME TO EXPLORE THE BODY CHEMISTRY ACTION PLAN?

➤ Have you worked through the Body Mechanics Action Plans but still have some lingering low-grade pain?

    ☐ Yes

    ☐ No

➤ Do you get relief from the Body Mechanics Action Plans, but your pain keeps returning?

    ☐ Yes

    ☐ No

➤ Do you also have any of the following:

    ☐ Minor digestive discomfort
       (bloating, heartburn, constipation, or loose stool)

    ☐ Headaches

    ☐ Minor upper respiratory symptoms (including postnasal drip)

    ☐ Skin rashes

    ☐ Other _____

If you answered "yes" to any or all of the above, it's a good time to explore this next section about body chemistry.

Notes:

_____

_____

_____

_____

_____

_____

_____

_____

_____

_____

_____

_____

_____

_____

_____

"In reality, a cell is a biological mini-me compared to the human body. A cell has every biological system that you have."

—Bruce Lipton

My *Release* Action Steps

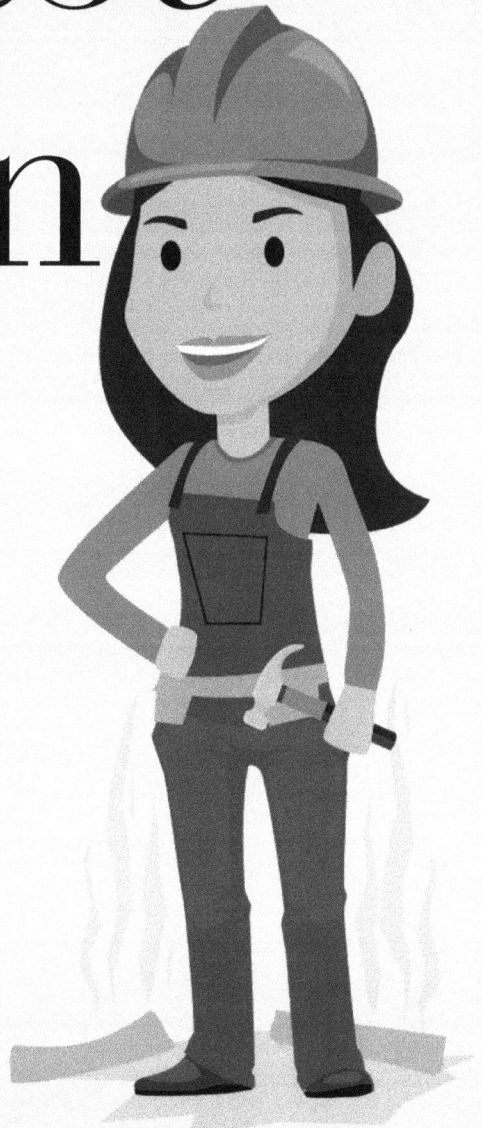

THE CHECK IN

How are you feeling?

TODAY'S DATE: _____

PAIN LOCATION:
(circle one)

Neck   Neck/Shoulder   Shoulder/Upper Back   Mid Back/Torso/Ribs

Low Back   Low Back/Hip   Hip/Buttock/Thigh

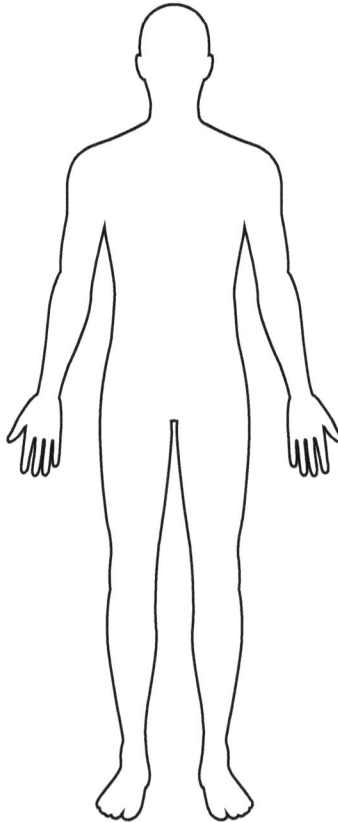

Use this figure to color or shade-in the area of your pain however you like.

HOW MUCH PAIN TODAY?

Circle the face below that best expresses your discomfort:

Wong-Baker FACES® Pain Rating Scale

0	2	4	6	8	10
No Pain	A Little Pain	A Little More Pain	Even More Pain	A Whole Lot Of Pain	Worst Pain

Notes:

_____

_____

_____

_____

_____

_____

_____

_____

_____

Digestion:
(circle all that apply)

Burping   Bloating   Passing gas   Belly pain

Constipation   Diarrhea/Loose stool

Other/More Details: _____

_____

_____

_____

_____

Breathing:
(circle all that apply)

Sniffly nose   Postnasal drip   Sinus congestion

Wheezing   Cough

Other/More Details: _____

_____

_____

_____

_____

Headaches:
(circle all that apply)

Forehead   Whole head   Right side   Left side

Other/More Details: _____

_____

_____

_____

_____

_____

Medication used:
(circle all that apply)

Inhaler   Antacids   Allergy tablets   Nasal spray/rinse

Ibuprofen (Motrin/Advil)   Naproxen (Aleve)

Aspirin   Acetaminophen (Tylenol)

Other/Prescription: _____

_____

How much? _____

_____

☐ Some Relief?   ☐ Total Relief?   ☐ No Relief?

RELEASE!

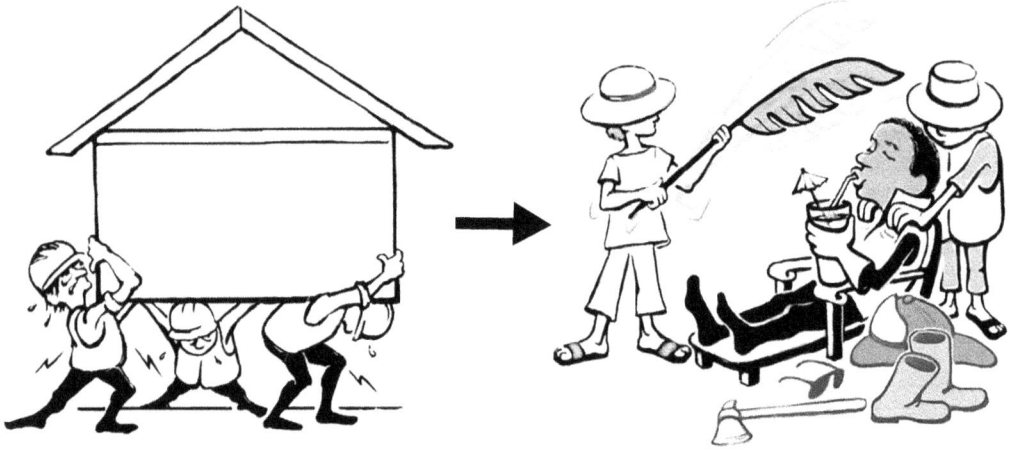

Q: *What* are you releasing?

A: **Poor quality or excess garbage-in**

Q: *How* are you releasing your poor quality or excess garbage-in?

A: **By identifying which of the big three and the sneaky three inflammation triggers are in your life. Then doing your best to take a break from as many as you can**

➤ Go to the book for more: *Fix the Fire Damage*, pages 398 – 426

➤ Listen to the podcast: *Conversations About Everyday Pain*, Season 2, Episodes 24 – 35

NEXT STEPS:

1. Release the **Big Three** triggers

2. Release your **Sneaky Three** triggers
   - Food sensitivities
   - Chemical sensitivities
   - Environmental allergies

3. Pick a maximum of three Release activities for daily use and record your progress in the following pages…

RELEASE THE BIG THREE

Pick one, two, or all three of the Big Three and pause your intake for 5-7 days while using a substitution.

- ➤ At the end of 5-7 days, how do you feel? Are you waking with less pain? How is your daytime body discomfort? Are you feeling more energy? Are you more tired but more relaxed?
- ➤ If things are going well, consider continuing to avoid or limit your big three intake as long as it continues to feel good.
- ➤ If you don't notice any difference but you're only decreasing intake, you may have to consider avoiding it completely.
- ➤ If you don't notice any difference and are completely avoiding one or two of the big three, you may have to switch to the next big three item(s) with a new 5-7 day trial of avoiding or decreasing intake of the one(s) that you haven't yet addressed.

RELEASE – WEEK 1

START DATE: _____

Check one to three of the following things to commit to changing/adding/pausing for the next 5-7 days.

Sugar Release

☐ Add Gymnema sylvestre or other blood sugar stabilizing nutrients (discuss with a professional)

☐ Increase foods high in fiber

☐ Focus on low glycemic index foods (refer to list at the back of this book)

☐ Decrease fruit and fruit juice intake

☐ Avoid artificial sweeteners in "sugar free" foods

Processed Foods Release

☐ Avoid packaged/processed foods and snacks

Caffeine Release

☐ Add B complex

☐ Morning workout

☐ Hearty breakfast

☐ Decaf alternatives: _____

☐ Adaptogens: (refer to back of the book for ideas)

REFLECTIONS

My current sources of high fiber foods:
(Visit pg 278 for high fiber food ideas.)

_____

_____

Foods I already eat that have a low glycemic index:
(Visit pg 276-277 for low glycemic index food ideas.)

_____

_____

Fruit and fruit juice intake that I can decrease:

_____

_____

"Sugar free" surprise sources of artificial sweeteners to avoid:

_____

_____

Foods in my diet with added fruit sugar:

_____

_____

NUTRIENT(S)/SUPPLEMENT(S) ADDED:

Food choices:

High fiber foods I choose this week:

_____

_____

Low glycemic index food choices:

_____

_____

Sources of fruit sugar that I skipped: (Yay me!)

_____

_____

Other foods:

_____

_____

_____

_____

_____

CRAVINGS

As you prepare for your week, circle your snack choices below based on your usual cravings:

Salty craving?
Mineral-rich food options:

Seaweed snacks   Nuts/Seeds   Shellfish   Eggs

Beans   Organ meats   Broccoli/Cauliflower

Other: _____

Rich/Fatty/Fried craving?
Health oils / Omega 3 foods:

Sardines   Salmon   Walnuts   Oysters   Edamame

Chia seeds   Flax   Anchovies   Mackerel

Other: _____

Hunger?
Lean protein ideas:

Plain Greek yogurt   Chicken breast   Turkey breast   Tofu

Grassfed beef   Beans   Lentils   Peas

Other: _____

Sweet craving?

High fiber foods:

Blueberries   Broccoli   Carrots (raw)   Avocado   Lentils

Beans   Artichoke hearts   Whole grain granola

Almonds   Pumpkin seeds

Other: _____

Craving comfort foods?

Take a nap!

Not sure what you're craving?

Hydrate!

Notes:

_____

_____

_____

_____

_____

_____

_____

TODAY'S DATE: _____

What was your body doing today?
(circle all that apply)

WORK

Sitting Standing Driving Repetitive Movement

Speaking Gig Phone Time Computer Time

Other: _____

PLAY

Roughhousing with young kids Tossing ball for the dog

Sitting on the floor

Other: _____

EXERCISE

Gym workout Swim Run Yoga Pilates

Bike (commute / stationary / trail)

Other: _____

Rate today's mood as well as your pain level:

Wong-Baker FACES® Pain Rating Scale

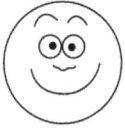 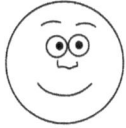 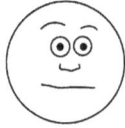 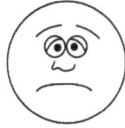 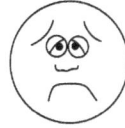 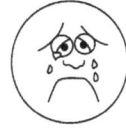

0	**2**	**4**	**6**	**8**	**10**
No Pain	A Little Pain	A Little More Pain	Even More Pain	A Whole Lot Of Pain	Worst Pain

How was your energy today?
(mark with an X)

SPUNKY   DRAGGING

Notes:

_____

_____

_____

_____

_____

_____

TODAY'S DATE: _____

What was your body doing today?
(circle all that apply)

WORK

Sitting   Standing   Driving   Repetitive Movement

Speaking Gig   Phone Time   Computer Time

Other: _____

PLAY

Roughhousing with young kids   Tossing ball for the dog

Sitting on the floor

Other: _____

EXERCISE

Gym workout   Swim   Run   Yoga   Pilates

Bike (commute / stationary / trail)

Other: _____

Rate today's mood as well as your pain level:

Wong-Baker FACES® Pain Rating Scale

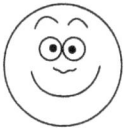 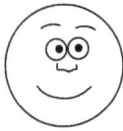 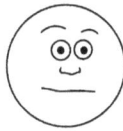 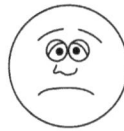 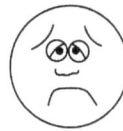 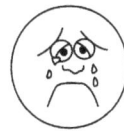

0	**2**	**4**	**6**	**8**	**10**
No Pain	A Little Pain	A Little More Pain	Even More Pain	A Whole Lot Of Pain	Worst Pain

How was your energy today?
(mark with an X)

SPUNKY   DRAGGING

Notes:

_____

_____

_____

_____

_____

_____

TODAY'S DATE: _____

What was your body doing today?
(circle all that apply)

WORK

Sitting   Standing   Driving   Repetitive Movement

Speaking Gig   Phone Time   Computer Time

Other: _____

PLAY

Roughhousing with young kids   Tossing ball for the dog

Sitting on the floor

Other: _____

EXERCISE

Gym workout   Swim   Run   Yoga   Pilates

Bike (commute / stationary / trail)

Other: _____

Rate today's mood as well as your pain level:

Wong-Baker FACES® Pain Rating Scale

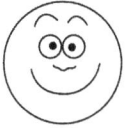 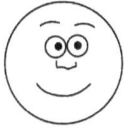 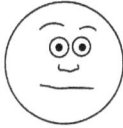 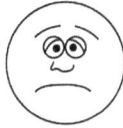 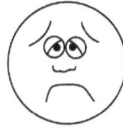 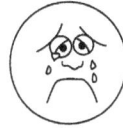

0	2	4	6	8	10
No Pain	A Little Pain	A Little More Pain	Even More Pain	A Whole Lot Of Pain	Worst Pain

How was your energy today?
(mark with an X)

SPUNKY

DRAGGING

Notes:

_____

_____

_____

_____

_____

_____

_____

TODAY'S DATE: _____

What was your body doing today?
(circle all that apply)

WORK

Sitting   Standing   Driving   Repetitive Movement

Speaking Gig   Phone Time   Computer Time

Other: _____

PLAY

Roughhousing with young kids   Tossing ball for the dog

Sitting on the floor

Other: _____

EXERCISE

Gym workout   Swim   Run   Yoga   Pilates

Bike (commute / stationary / trail)

Other: _____

Rate today's mood as well as your pain level:

Wong-Baker FACES® Pain Rating Scale

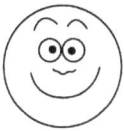 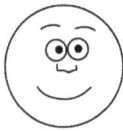 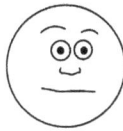 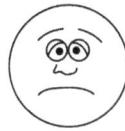 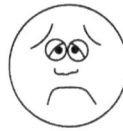 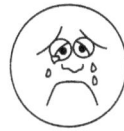

0	2	4	6	8	10
No Pain	A Little Pain	A Little More Pain	Even More Pain	A Whole Lot Of Pain	Worst Pain

How was your energy today?
(mark with an X)

SPUNKY   DRAGGING

Notes:

_____

_____

_____

_____

_____

_____

_____

TODAY'S DATE: _____

What was your body doing today?
(circle all that apply)

WORK

Sitting   Standing   Driving   Repetitive Movement

Speaking Gig   Phone Time   Computer Time

Other: _____

PLAY

Roughhousing with young kids   Tossing ball for the dog

Sitting on the floor

Other: _____

EXERCISE

Gym workout   Swim   Run   Yoga   Pilates

Bike (commute / stationary / trail)

Other: _____

Rate today's mood as well as your pain level:

Wong-Baker FACES® Pain Rating Scale

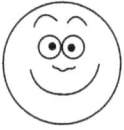 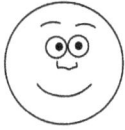 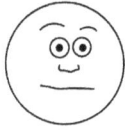 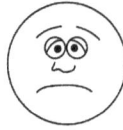 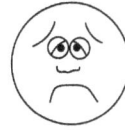 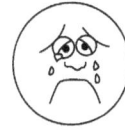

0	2	4	6	8	10
No Pain	A Little Pain	A Little More Pain	Even More Pain	A Whole Lot Of Pain	Worst Pain

How was your energy today?
(mark with an X)

SPUNKY   DRAGGING

Notes:

_____

_____

_____

_____

_____

_____

TODAY'S DATE: _____

What was your body doing today?
(circle all that apply)

WORK

Sitting Standing Driving Repetitive Movement

Speaking Gig Phone Time Computer Time

Other: _____

PLAY

Roughhousing with young kids Tossing ball for the dog

Sitting on the floor

Other: _____

EXERCISE

Gym workout Swim Run Yoga Pilates

Bike (commute / stationary / trail)

Other: _____

Rate today's mood as well as your pain level:

Wong-Baker FACES® Pain Rating Scale

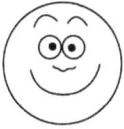 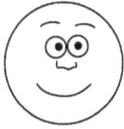 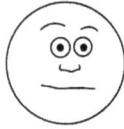 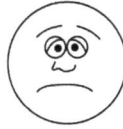 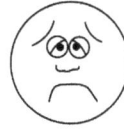 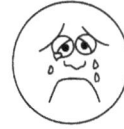

0	**2**	**4**	**6**	**8**	**10**
No Pain	A Little Pain	A Little More Pain	Even More Pain	A Whole Lot Of Pain	Worst Pain

How was your energy today?
(mark with an X)

SPUNKY   DRAGGING

Notes:

_____

_____

_____

_____

_____

_____

_____

TODAY'S DATE: _____

What was your body doing today?
(circle all that apply)

WORK

Sitting   Standing   Driving   Repetitive Movement

Speaking Gig   Phone Time   Computer Time

Other: _____

PLAY

Roughhousing with young kids   Tossing ball for the dog

Sitting on the floor

Other: _____

EXERCISE

Gym workout   Swim   Run   Yoga   Pilates

Bike (commute / stationary / trail)

Other: _____

Rate today's mood as well as your pain level:

Wong-Baker FACES® Pain Rating Scale

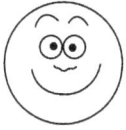 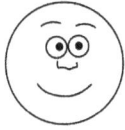 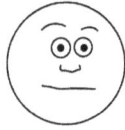 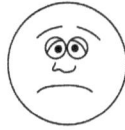 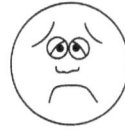 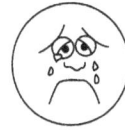

0	2	4	6	8	10
No Pain	A Little Pain	A Little More Pain	Even More Pain	A Whole Lot Of Pain	Worst Pain

How was your energy today?
(mark with an X)

SPUNKY   DRAGGING

Notes:

_____

_____

_____

_____

_____

_____

_____

YOU MADE IT TO THE END OF WEEK 1!

How are you feeling?

TODAY'S DATE: _____

PAIN LOCATION:
(circle one)

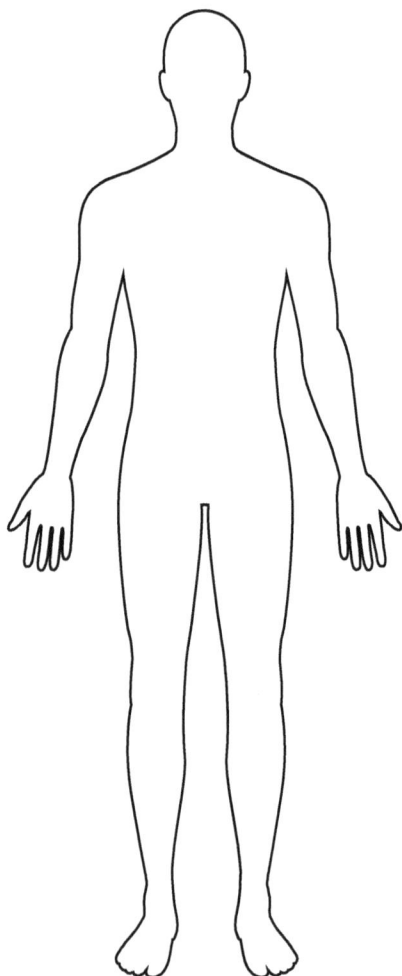

Neck

Neck/Shoulder

Shoulder/Upper Back

Mid Back/Torso/Ribs

Low Back

Low Back/Hip

Hip/Buttock/Thigh

Use this figure to color or shade-in the area of your pain however you like.

HOW MUCH PAIN TODAY?

Circle the face below that best expresses your discomfort:

Wong-Baker FACES® Pain Rating Scale

0	2	4	6	8	10
No Pain	A Little Pain	A Little More Pain	Even More Pain	A Whole Lot Of Pain	Worst Pain

Notes:

_____

_____

_____

_____

_____

_____

_____

_____

_____

RELEASE – WEEK 1

Digestion:
(circle all that apply)

Burping   Bloating   Passing gas   Belly pain

Constipation   Diarrhea/Loose stool

Other/More Details: _____

_____

_____

_____

_____

Breathing:
(circle all that apply)

Sniffly nose   Postnasal drip   Sinus congestion

Wheezing   Cough

Other/More Details: _____

_____

_____

_____

_____

Headaches:
(circle all that apply)

Forehead   Whole head   Right side   Left side

Other/More Details: _____

_____

_____

_____

_____

_____

Medication used:
(circle all that apply)

Inhaler   Antacids   Allergy tablets   Nasal spray/rinse

Ibuprofen (Motrin/Advil)   Naproxen (Aleve)

Aspirin   Acetaminophen (Tylenol)

Other/Prescription: _____

_____

How much? _____

_____

☐ Some Relief?   ☐ Total Relief?   ☐ No Relief?

REFLECTIONS

What worked? / What didn't work? Think about next steps: continue or try pausing one of the other Big Three triggers...

_____

_____

_____

_____

_____

_____

_____

_____

_____

_____

_____

_____

_____

AFFIRMATION:

Repeat out loud:

"I will feel calmer and less inflamed every day without sugar hijacking my brain."

AFFIRMATION:

Repeat out loud:

"My food cravings come from my body's wisdom. I welcome and honor the information."

RELEASE - WEEK 2

START DATE: _____

Check one to three of the following things to commit to changing/adding/pausing for the next 5-7 days.

Sugar Release

☐ Add Gymnema sylvestre or other blood sugar stabilizing nutrients (discuss with a professional)

☐ Increase foods high in fiber

☐ Focus on low glycemic index foods (refer to list at the back of this book)

☐ Decrease fruit and fruit juice intake

☐ Avoid artificial sweeteners in "sugar free" foods

Processed Foods Release

☐ Avoid packaged/processed foods and snacks

Caffeine Release

☐ Add B complex

☐ Morning workout

☐ Hearty breakfast

☐ Decaf alternatives: _____

☐ Adaptogens: (refer to back of the book for ideas)

REFLECTIONS

My current sources of high fiber foods:
(Visit pg 278 for high fiber food ideas.)

_____

_____

Foods I already eat that have a low glycemic index:
(Visit pg 276-277 for low glycemic index food ideas.)

_____

_____

Fruit and fruit juice intake that I can decrease:

_____

_____

"Sugar free" surprise sources of artificial sweeteners to avoid:

_____

_____

Foods in my diet with added fruit sugar:

_____

_____

NUTRIENT(S)/SUPPLEMENT(S) ADDED:

Food choices:
High fiber foods I choose this week:

_____

_____

Low glycemic index food choices:

_____

_____

Sources of fruit sugar that I skipped: (Yay me!)

_____

_____

Other foods:

_____

_____

_____

_____

_____

_____

CRAVINGS

As you prepare for your week, circle your snack choices below based on your usual cravings:

Salty craving?

Mineral-rich food options:

Seaweed snacks   Nuts/Seeds   Shellfish   Eggs

Beans   Organ meats   Broccoli/Cauliflower

Other: _____

Rich/Fatty/Fried craving?

Health oils / Omega 3 foods:

Sardines   Salmon   Walnuts   Oysters   Edamame

Chia seeds   Flax   Anchovies   Mackerel

Other: _____

Hunger?

Lean protein ideas:

Plain Greek yogurt   Chicken breast   Turkey breast   Tofu

Grassfed beef   Beans   Lentils   Peas

Other: _____

Sweet craving?

High fiber foods:

Blueberries   Broccoli   Carrots (raw)   Avocado   Lentils

Beans   Artichoke hearts   Whole grain granola

Almonds   Pumpkin seeds

Other: _____

Craving comfort foods?

Take a nap!

Not sure what you're craving?

Hydrate!

Notes:

_____

_____

_____

_____

_____

_____

_____

_____

TODAY'S DATE: _____

What was your body doing today?
(circle all that apply)

WORK

Sitting   Standing   Driving   Repetitive Movement

Speaking Gig   Phone Time   Computer Time

Other: _____

PLAY

Roughhousing with young kids   Tossing ball for the dog

Sitting on the floor

Other: _____

EXERCISE

Gym workout   Swim   Run   Yoga   Pilates

Bike (commute / stationary / trail)

Other: _____

Rate today's mood as well as your pain level:

Wong-Baker FACES® Pain Rating Scale

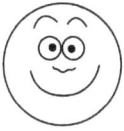 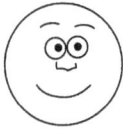 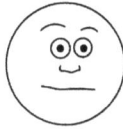 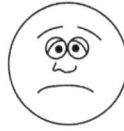 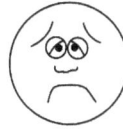 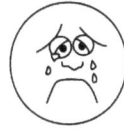

0	**2**	**4**	**6**	**8**	**10**
No Pain	A Little Pain	A Little More Pain	Even More Pain	A Whole Lot Of Pain	Worst Pain

How was your energy today?
(mark with an X)

SPUNKY   DRAGGING

Notes:

_____

_____

_____

_____

_____

_____

TODAY'S DATE: _____

What was your body doing today?
(circle all that apply)

WORK

Sitting   Standing   Driving   Repetitive Movement

Speaking Gig   Phone Time   Computer Time

Other: _____

PLAY

Roughhousing with young kids   Tossing ball for the dog

Sitting on the floor

Other: _____

EXERCISE

Gym workout   Swim   Run   Yoga   Pilates

Bike (commute / stationary / trail)

Other: _____

Rate today's mood as well as your pain level:

Wong-Baker FACES® Pain Rating Scale

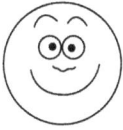 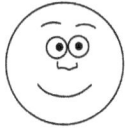 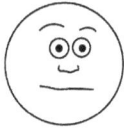 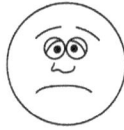 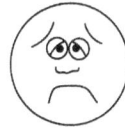 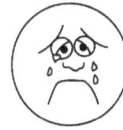

0	**2**	**4**	**6**	**8**	**10**
No Pain	A Little Pain	A Little More Pain	Even More Pain	A Whole Lot Of Pain	Worst Pain

How was your energy today?
(mark with an X)

SPUNKY   DRAGGING

Notes:

_____

_____

_____

_____

_____

_____

_____

TODAY'S DATE: _____

What was your body doing today?
(circle all that apply)

WORK

Sitting   Standing   Driving   Repetitive Movement

Speaking Gig   Phone Time   Computer Time

Other: _____

PLAY

Roughhousing with young kids   Tossing ball for the dog

Sitting on the floor

Other: _____

EXERCISE

Gym workout   Swim   Run   Yoga   Pilates

Bike (commute / stationary / trail)

Other: _____

Rate today's mood as well as your pain level:

Wong-Baker FACES® Pain Rating Scale

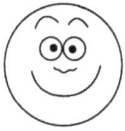 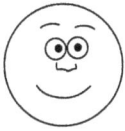 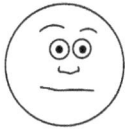 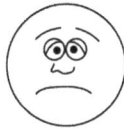 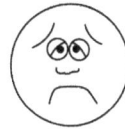 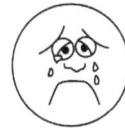

0	**2**	**4**	**6**	**8**	**10**
No Pain	A Little Pain	A Little More Pain	Even More Pain	A Whole Lot Of Pain	Worst Pain

How was your energy today?
(mark with an X)

SPUNKY   DRAGGING

Notes:

_____

_____

_____

_____

_____

_____

TODAY'S DATE: _____

What was your body doing today?
(circle all that apply)

WORK

Sitting   Standing   Driving   Repetitive Movement

Speaking Gig   Phone Time   Computer Time

Other: _____

PLAY

Roughhousing with young kids   Tossing ball for the dog

Sitting on the floor

Other: _____

EXERCISE

Gym workout   Swim   Run   Yoga   Pilates

Bike (commute / stationary / trail)

Other: _____

Rate today's mood as well as your pain level:

Wong-Baker FACES® Pain Rating Scale

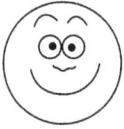 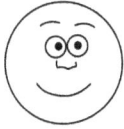 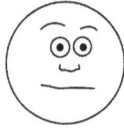 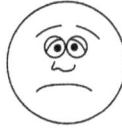 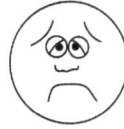 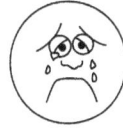

0	2	4	6	8	10
No Pain	A Little Pain	A Little More Pain	Even More Pain	A Whole Lot Of Pain	Worst Pain

How was your energy today?
(mark with an X)

SPUNKY   DRAGGING

Notes:

_____

_____

_____

_____

_____

_____

_____

TODAY'S DATE: _____

What was your body doing today?
(circle all that apply)

WORK

Sitting   Standing   Driving   Repetitive Movement

Speaking Gig   Phone Time   Computer Time

Other: _____

PLAY

Roughhousing with young kids   Tossing ball for the dog

Sitting on the floor

Other: _____

EXERCISE

Gym workout   Swim   Run   Yoga   Pilates

Bike (commute / stationary / trail)

Other: _____

Rate today's mood as well as your pain level:

Wong-Baker FACES® Pain Rating Scale

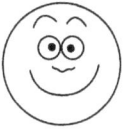 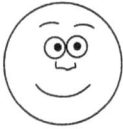 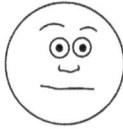 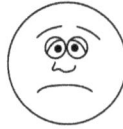 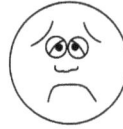 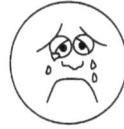

0	**2**	**4**	**6**	**8**	**10**
No Pain	A Little Pain	A Little More Pain	Even More Pain	A Whole Lot Of Pain	Worst Pain

How was your energy today?
(mark with an X)

SPUNKY   DRAGGING

Notes:

_____

_____

_____

_____

_____

_____

TODAY'S DATE: _____

What was your body doing today?
(circle all that apply)

WORK

Sitting   Standing   Driving   Repetitive Movement

Speaking Gig   Phone Time   Computer Time

Other: _____

PLAY

Roughhousing with young kids   Tossing ball for the dog

Sitting on the floor

Other: _____

EXERCISE

Gym workout   Swim   Run   Yoga   Pilates

Bike (commute / stationary / trail)

Other: _____

Rate today's mood as well as your pain level:

Wong-Baker FACES® Pain Rating Scale

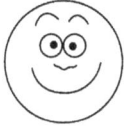 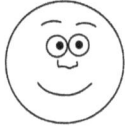 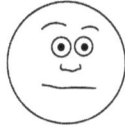 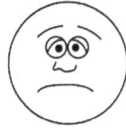 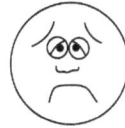 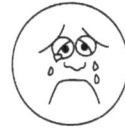

0	2	4	6	8	10
No Pain	A Little Pain	A Little More Pain	Even More Pain	A Whole Lot Of Pain	Worst Pain

How was your energy today?
(mark with an X)

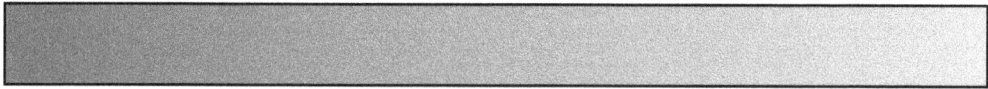

SPUNKY   DRAGGING

Notes:

_____

_____

_____

_____

_____

_____

_____

TODAY'S DATE: _____

What was your body doing today?
(circle all that apply)

WORK

Sitting   Standing   Driving   Repetitive Movement

Speaking Gig   Phone Time   Computer Time

Other: _____

PLAY

Roughhousing with young kids   Tossing ball for the dog

Sitting on the floor

Other: _____

EXERCISE

Gym workout   Swim   Run   Yoga   Pilates

Bike (commute / stationary / trail)

Other: _____

Rate today's mood as well as your pain level:

Wong-Baker FACES® Pain Rating Scale

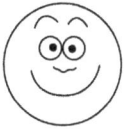 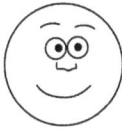 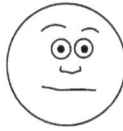 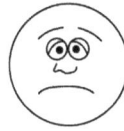 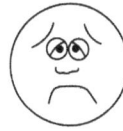 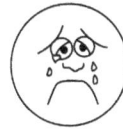

0	**2**	**4**	**6**	**8**	**10**
No Pain	A Little Pain	A Little More Pain	Even More Pain	A Whole Lot Of Pain	Worst Pain

How was your energy today?
(mark with an X)

SPUNKY   DRAGGING

Notes:

_____

_____

_____

_____

_____

_____

YOU MADE IT TO THE END OF WEEK 2!

How are you feeling?

TODAY'S DATE: _____

PAIN LOCATION:
(circle one)

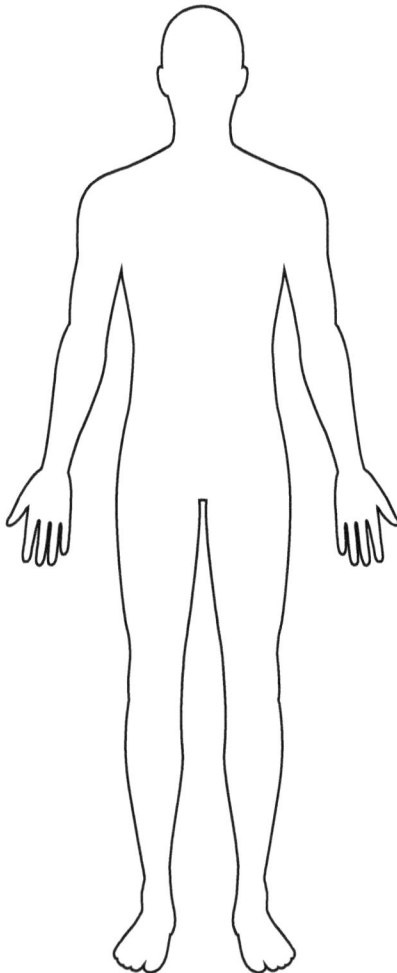

Neck

Neck/Shoulder

Shoulder/Upper Back

Mid Back/Torso/Ribs

Low Back

Low Back/Hip

Hip/Buttock/Thigh

Use this figure to color or shade-in the area of your pain however you like.

HOW MUCH PAIN TODAY?

Circle the face below that best expresses your discomfort:

Wong-Baker FACES® Pain Rating Scale

0	2	4	6	8	10
No Pain	A Little Pain	A Little More Pain	Even More Pain	A Whole Lot Of Pain	Worst Pain

Notes:

_____

_____

_____

_____

_____

_____

_____

_____

_____

Digestion:
(circle all that apply)

Burping   Bloating   Passing gas   Belly pain

Constipation   Diarrhea/Loose stool

Other/More Details: _____

_____

_____

_____

_____

Breathing:
(circle all that apply)

Sniffly nose   Postnasal drip   Sinus congestion

Wheezing   Cough

Other/More Details: _____

_____

_____

_____

_____

Headaches:
(circle all that apply)

Forehead   Whole head   Right side   Left side

Other/More Details: _____

_____

_____

_____

_____

Medication used:
(circle all that apply)

Inhaler   Antacids   Allergy tablets   Nasal spray/rinse

Ibuprofen (Motrin/Advil)   Naproxen (Aleve)

Aspirin   Acetaminophen (Tylenol)

Other/Prescription: _____

_____

How much? _____

_____

☐ Some Relief?   ☐ Total Relief?   ☐ No Relief?

REFLECTIONS

What worked? / What didn't work? Think about next steps: continue or try pausing one of the other Big Three triggers…

_____

_____

_____

_____

_____

_____

_____

_____

_____

_____

_____

_____

_____

AFFIRMATION:

Repeat out loud:

"I am naturally energized – no coffee beans needed."

AFFIRMATION:

Repeat out loud:

"My body

thanks me

for choosing

rest over

rocket fuel!"

RELEASE - WEEK 3

START DATE: _____

Check one to three of the following things to commit to changing/adding/pausing for the next 5-7 days.

Sugar Release

☐ Add Gymnema sylvestre or other blood sugar stabilizing nutrients (discuss with a professional)

☐ Increase foods high in fiber

☐ Focus on low glycemic index foods (refer to list at the back of this book)

☐ Decrease fruit and fruit juice intake

☐ Avoid artificial sweeteners in "sugar free" foods

Processed Foods Release

☐ Avoid packaged/processed foods and snacks

Caffeine Release

☐ Add B complex

☐ Morning workout

☐ Hearty breakfast

☐ Decaf alternatives: _____

☐ Adaptogens: (refer to back of the book for ideas)

REFLECTIONS

My current sources of high fiber foods:
(Visit pg 278 for high fiber food ideas.)

_____

_____

Foods I already eat that have a low glycemic index:
(Visit pg 276-277 for low glycemic index food ideas.)

_____

_____

Fruit and fruit juice intake that I can decrease:

_____

_____

"Sugar free" surprise sources of artificial sweeteners to avoid:

_____

_____

Foods in my diet with added fruit sugar:

_____

_____

NUTRIENT(S)/SUPPLEMENT(S) ADDED:

Food choices:

High fiber foods I choose this week:

_____

_____

Low glycemic index food choices:

_____

_____

Sources of fruit sugar that I skipped: (Yay me!)

_____

_____

Other foods:

_____

_____

_____

_____

_____

_____

CRAVINGS

As you prepare for your week, circle your snack choices below based on your usual cravings:

Salty craving?
Mineral-rich food options:

Seaweed snacks   Nuts/Seeds   Shellfish   Eggs

Beans   Organ meats   Broccoli/Cauliflower

Other: _____

Rich/Fatty/Fried craving?
Health oils / Omega 3 foods:

Sardines   Salmon   Walnuts   Oysters   Edamame

Chia seeds   Flax   Anchovies   Mackerel

Other: _____

Hunger?
Lean protein ideas:

Plain Greek yogurt   Chicken breast   Turkey breast   Tofu

Grassfed beef   Beans   Lentils   Peas

Other: _____

Sweet craving?

High fiber foods:

Blueberries   Broccoli   Carrots (raw)   Avocado   Lentils

Beans   Artichoke hearts   Whole grain granola

Almonds   Pumpkin seeds

Other: _____

Craving comfort foods?

Take a nap!

Not sure what you're craving?

Hydrate!

Notes:

_____

_____

_____

_____

_____

_____

_____

TODAY'S DATE: _____

What was your body doing today?
(circle all that apply)

WORK

Sitting   Standing   Driving   Repetitive Movement

Speaking Gig   Phone Time   Computer Time

Other: _____

PLAY

Roughhousing with young kids   Tossing ball for the dog

Sitting on the floor

Other: _____

EXERCISE

Gym workout   Swim   Run   Yoga   Pilates

Bike (commute / stationary / trail)

Other: _____

Rate today's mood as well as your pain level:

Wong-Baker FACES® Pain Rating Scale

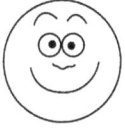 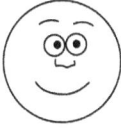 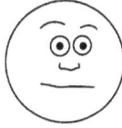 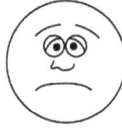 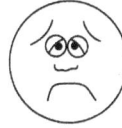 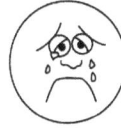

0	**2**	**4**	**6**	**8**	**10**
No Pain	A Little Pain	A Little More Pain	Even More Pain	A Whole Lot Of Pain	Worst Pain

How was your energy today?
(mark with an X)

SPUNKY   DRAGGING

Notes:

_____

_____

_____

_____

_____

_____

TODAY'S DATE: _____

What was your body doing today?
(circle all that apply)

WORK

Sitting   Standing   Driving   Repetitive Movement

Speaking Gig   Phone Time   Computer Time

Other: _____

PLAY

Roughhousing with young kids   Tossing ball for the dog

Sitting on the floor

Other: _____

EXERCISE

Gym workout   Swim   Run   Yoga   Pilates

Bike (commute / stationary / trail)

Other: _____

Rate today's mood as well as your pain level:

Wong-Baker FACES® Pain Rating Scale

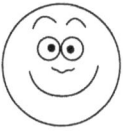 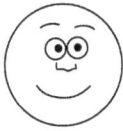 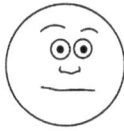 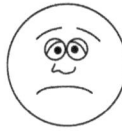 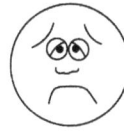 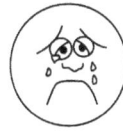

0	**2**	**4**	**6**	**8**	**10**
No Pain	A Little Pain	A Little More Pain	Even More Pain	A Whole Lot Of Pain	Worst Pain

How was your energy today?
(mark with an X)

SPUNKY   DRAGGING

Notes:

_____

_____

_____

_____

_____

_____

TODAY'S DATE: _____

What was your body doing today?
(circle all that apply)

WORK

Sitting   Standing   Driving   Repetitive Movement

Speaking Gig   Phone Time   Computer Time

Other: _____

PLAY

Roughhousing with young kids   Tossing ball for the dog

Sitting on the floor

Other: _____

EXERCISE

Gym workout   Swim   Run   Yoga   Pilates

Bike (commute / stationary / trail)

Other: _____

Rate today's mood as well as your pain level:

Wong-Baker FACES® Pain Rating Scale

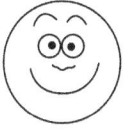 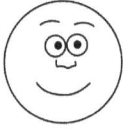 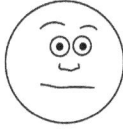 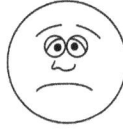 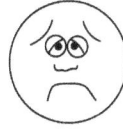 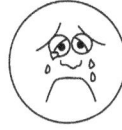

0	**2**	**4**	**6**	**8**	**10**
No Pain	A Little Pain	A Little More Pain	Even More Pain	A Whole Lot Of Pain	Worst Pain

How was your energy today?
(mark with an X)

SPUNKY   DRAGGING

Notes:

_____

_____

_____

_____

_____

_____

TODAY'S DATE: _____

What was your body doing today?
(circle all that apply)

WORK

Sitting   Standing   Driving   Repetitive Movement

Speaking Gig   Phone Time   Computer Time

Other: _____

PLAY

Roughhousing with young kids   Tossing ball for the dog

Sitting on the floor

Other: _____

EXERCISE

Gym workout   Swim   Run   Yoga   Pilates

Bike (commute / stationary / trail)

Other: _____

Rate today's mood as well as your pain level:

Wong-Baker FACES® Pain Rating Scale

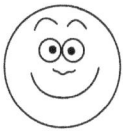 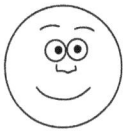 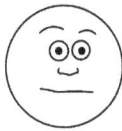 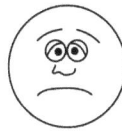 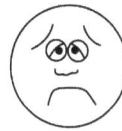 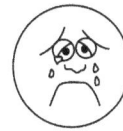

0	2	4	6	8	10
No Pain	A Little Pain	A Little More Pain	Even More Pain	A Whole Lot Of Pain	Worst Pain

How was your energy today?
(mark with an X)

SPUNKY   DRAGGING

Notes:

_____

_____

_____

_____

_____

_____

TODAY'S DATE: _____

What was your body doing today?
(circle all that apply)

WORK

Sitting   Standing   Driving   Repetitive Movement

Speaking Gig   Phone Time   Computer Time

Other: _____

PLAY

Roughhousing with young kids   Tossing ball for the dog

Sitting on the floor

Other: _____

EXERCISE

Gym workout   Swim   Run   Yoga   Pilates

Bike (commute / stationary / trail)

Other: _____

Rate today's mood as well as your pain level:

Wong-Baker FACES® Pain Rating Scale

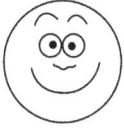 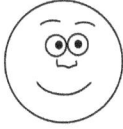 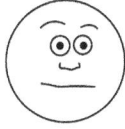 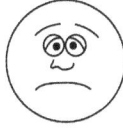 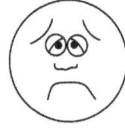 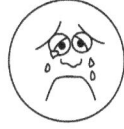

0	**2**	**4**	**6**	**8**	**10**
No Pain	A Little Pain	A Little More Pain	Even More Pain	A Whole Lot Of Pain	Worst Pain

How was your energy today?
(mark with an X)

SPUNKY   DRAGGING

Notes:

_____

_____

_____

_____

_____

_____

TODAY'S DATE: _____

What was your body doing today?
(circle all that apply)

WORK

Sitting   Standing   Driving   Repetitive Movement

Speaking Gig   Phone Time   Computer Time

Other: _____

PLAY

Roughhousing with young kids   Tossing ball for the dog

Sitting on the floor

Other: _____

EXERCISE

Gym workout   Swim   Run   Yoga   Pilates

Bike (commute / stationary / trail)

Other: _____

Rate today's mood as well as your pain level:

Wong-Baker FACES® Pain Rating Scale

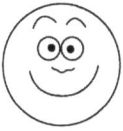 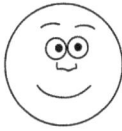 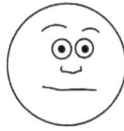 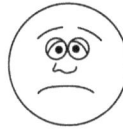 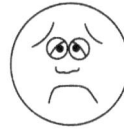 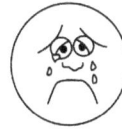

0	2	4	6	8	10
No Pain	A Little Pain	A Little More Pain	Even More Pain	A Whole Lot Of Pain	Worst Pain

How was your energy today?
(mark with an X)

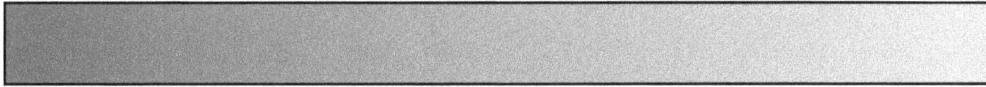

SPUNKY   DRAGGING

Notes:

_____

_____

_____

_____

_____

_____

TODAY'S DATE: _____

What was your body doing today?
(circle all that apply)

WORK

Sitting   Standing   Driving   Repetitive Movement

Speaking Gig   Phone Time   Computer Time

Other: _____

PLAY

Roughhousing with young kids   Tossing ball for the dog

Sitting on the floor

Other: _____

EXERCISE

Gym workout   Swim   Run   Yoga   Pilates

Bike (commute / stationary / trail)

Other: _____

Rate today's mood as well as your pain level:

Wong-Baker FACES® Pain Rating Scale

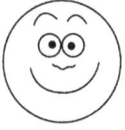 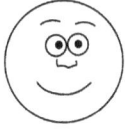 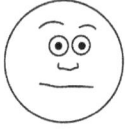 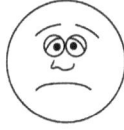 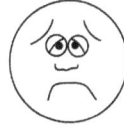 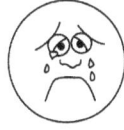

0	**2**	**4**	**6**	**8**	**10**
No Pain	A Little Pain	A Little More Pain	Even More Pain	A Whole Lot Of Pain	Worst Pain

How was your energy today?
(mark with an X)

SPUNKY   DRAGGING

Notes:

_____

_____

_____

_____

_____

_____

_____

YOU MADE IT TO THE END OF WEEK 3!

How are you feeling?

TODAY'S DATE: _____

PAIN LOCATION:
(circle one)

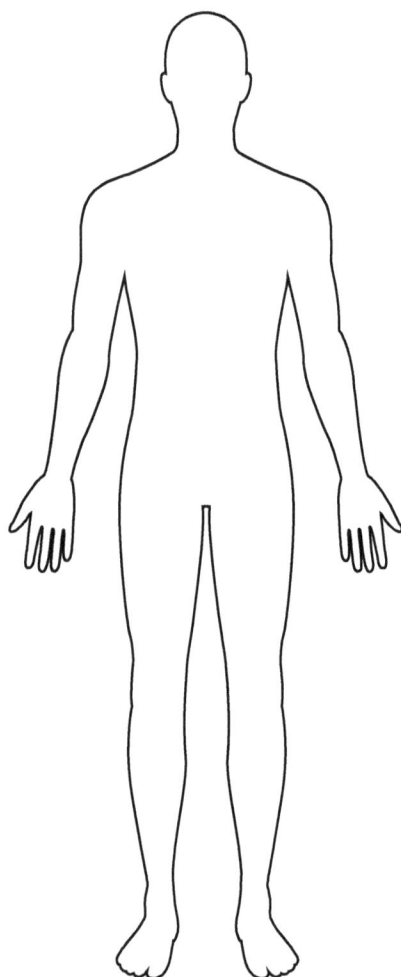

Neck

Neck/Shoulder

Shoulder/Upper Back

Mid Back/Torso/Ribs

Low Back

Low Back/Hip

Hip/Buttock/Thigh

Use this figure to color or shade-in the area of your pain however you like.

HOW MUCH PAIN TODAY?

Circle the face below that best expresses your discomfort:

Wong-Baker FACES® Pain Rating Scale

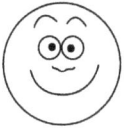 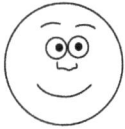 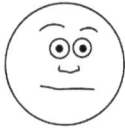 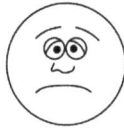 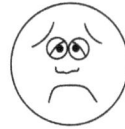 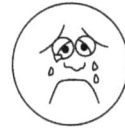

0	2	4	6	8	10
No Pain	A Little Pain	A Little More Pain	Even More Pain	A Whole Lot Of Pain	Worst Pain

Notes:

_____

_____

_____

_____

_____

_____

_____

_____

_____

RELEASE - WEEK 3

Digestion:
(circle all that apply)

Burping   Bloating   Passing gas   Belly pain

Constipation   Diarrhea/Loose stool

Other/More Details: _____

_____

_____

_____

_____

Breathing:
(circle all that apply)

Sniffly nose   Postnasal drip   Sinus congestion

Wheezing   Cough

Other/More Details: _____

_____

_____

_____

_____

Headaches:
(circle all that apply)

Forehead   Whole head   Right side   Left side

Other/More Details: _____

_____

_____

_____

_____

Medication used:
(circle all that apply)

Inhaler   Antacids   Allergy tablets   Nasal spray/rinse

Ibuprofen (Motrin/Advil)   Naproxen (Aleve)

Aspirin   Acetaminophen (Tylenol)

Other/Prescription: _____

_____

How much? _____

_____

☐ Some Relief?   ☐ Total Relief?   ☐ No Relief?

REFLECTIONS

What worked? / What didn't work? Think about next steps: continue or try pausing one of the other Big Three triggers...

_____

_____

_____

_____

_____

_____

_____

_____

_____

_____

_____

_____

_____

AFFIRMATION:

Repeat out loud:

"By letting go of sugar, I am making space for more energy, clarity, and balance."

AFFIRMATION:

Repeat out loud:

"I will nourish my body with wholesome, natural foods that feed my vibrancy."

RELEASE - WEEK 4

START DATE: _____

Check one to three of the following things to commit to changing/adding/pausing for the next 5-7 days.

Sugar Release

☐ Add Gymnema sylvestre or other blood sugar stabilizing nutrients (discuss with a professional)

☐ Increase foods high in fiber

☐ Focus on low glycemic index foods (refer to list at the back of this book)

☐ Decrease fruit and fruit juice intake

☐ Avoid artificial sweeteners in "sugar free" foods

Processed Foods Release

☐ Avoid packaged/processed foods and snacks

Caffeine Release

☐ Add B complex

☐ Morning workout

☐ Hearty breakfast

☐ Decaf alternatives: _____

☐ Adaptogens: (refer to back of the book for ideas)

REFLECTIONS

My current sources of high fiber foods:
(Visit pg 278 for high fiber food ideas.)

_____

_____

Foods I already eat that have a low glycemic index:
(Visit pg 276-277 for low glycemic index food ideas.)

_____

_____

Fruit and fruit juice intake that I can decrease:

_____

_____

"Sugar free" surprise sources of artificial sweeteners to avoid:

_____

_____

Foods in my diet with added fruit sugar:

_____

_____

NUTRIENT(S)/SUPPLEMENT(S) ADDED:

Food choices:

High fiber foods I choose this week:

_____

_____

Low glycemic index food choices:

_____

_____

Sources of fruit sugar that I skipped: (Yay me!)

_____

_____

Other foods:

_____

_____

_____

_____

_____

CRAVINGS

As you prepare for your week, circle your snack choices below based on your usual cravings:

Salty craving?
Mineral-rich food options:

Seaweed snacks   Nuts/Seeds   Shellfish   Eggs

Beans   Organ meats   Broccoli/Cauliflower

Other: _____

Rich/Fatty/Fried craving?
Health oils / Omega 3 foods:

Sardines   Salmon   Walnuts   Oysters   Edamame

Chia seeds   Flax   Anchovies   Mackerel

Other: _____

Hunger?
Lean protein ideas:

Plain Greek yogurt   Chicken breast   Turkey breast   Tofu

Grassfed beef   Beans   Lentils   Peas

Other: _____

Sweet craving?

High fiber foods:

Blueberries   Broccoli   Carrots (raw)   Avocado   Lentils

Beans   Artichoke hearts   Whole grain granola

Almonds   Pumpkin seeds

Other: _____

Craving comfort foods?

Take a nap!

Not sure what you're craving?

Hydrate!

Notes:

_____

_____

_____

_____

_____

_____

_____

TODAY'S DATE: _____

What was your body doing today?
(circle all that apply)

WORK

Sitting   Standing   Driving   Repetitive Movement

Speaking Gig   Phone Time   Computer Time

Other: _____

PLAY

Roughhousing with young kids   Tossing ball for the dog

Sitting on the floor

Other: _____

EXERCISE

Gym workout   Swim   Run   Yoga   Pilates

Bike (commute / stationary / trail)

Other: _____

Rate today's mood as well as your pain level:

Wong-Baker FACES® Pain Rating Scale

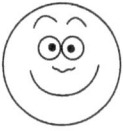 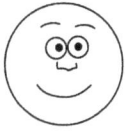 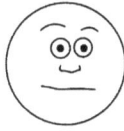 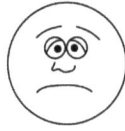 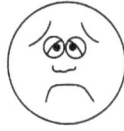 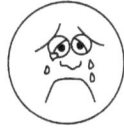

0	2	4	6	8	10
No Pain	A Little Pain	A Little More Pain	Even More Pain	A Whole Lot Of Pain	Worst Pain

How was your energy today?
(mark with an X)

SPUNKY   DRAGGING

Notes:

_____

_____

_____

_____

_____

_____

TODAY'S DATE: _____

What was your body doing today?
(circle all that apply)

WORK

Sitting   Standing   Driving   Repetitive Movement

Speaking Gig   Phone Time   Computer Time

Other: _____

PLAY

Roughhousing with young kids   Tossing ball for the dog

Sitting on the floor

Other: _____

EXERCISE

Gym workout   Swim   Run   Yoga   Pilates

Bike (commute / stationary / trail)

Other: _____

Rate today's mood as well as your pain level:

Wong-Baker FACES® Pain Rating Scale

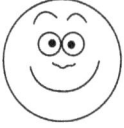 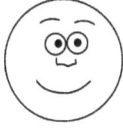 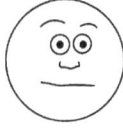 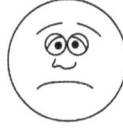 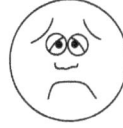 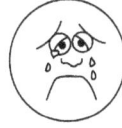

0	2	4	6	8	10
No Pain	A Little Pain	A Little More Pain	Even More Pain	A Whole Lot Of Pain	Worst Pain

How was your energy today?
(mark with an X)

SPUNKY   DRAGGING

Notes:

_____

_____

_____

_____

_____

_____

_____

TODAY'S DATE: _____

What was your body doing today?
(circle all that apply)

WORK

Sitting   Standing   Driving   Repetitive Movement

Speaking Gig   Phone Time   Computer Time

Other: _____

PLAY

Roughhousing with young kids   Tossing ball for the dog

Sitting on the floor

Other: _____

EXERCISE

Gym workout   Swim   Run   Yoga   Pilates

Bike (commute / stationary / trail)

Other: _____

Rate today's mood as well as your pain level:

Wong-Baker FACES® Pain Rating Scale

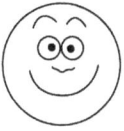 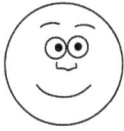 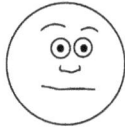 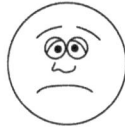 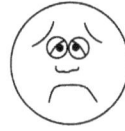 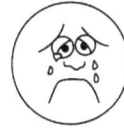

0	**2**	**4**	**6**	**8**	**10**
No Pain	A Little Pain	A Little More Pain	Even More Pain	A Whole Lot Of Pain	Worst Pain

How was your energy today?
(mark with an X)

SPUNKY   DRAGGING

Notes:

_____

_____

_____

_____

_____

_____

TODAY'S DATE: _____

What was your body doing today?
(circle all that apply)

WORK

Sitting   Standing   Driving   Repetitive Movement

Speaking Gig   Phone Time   Computer Time

Other: _____

PLAY

Roughhousing with young kids   Tossing ball for the dog

Sitting on the floor

Other: _____

EXERCISE

Gym workout   Swim   Run   Yoga   Pilates

Bike (commute / stationary / trail)

Other: _____

Rate today's mood as well as your pain level:

Wong-Baker FACES® Pain Rating Scale

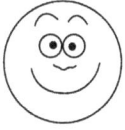 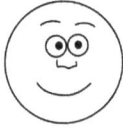 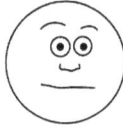 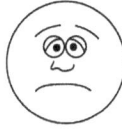 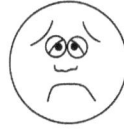 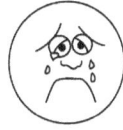

0	**2**	**4**	**6**	**8**	**10**
No Pain	A Little Pain	A Little More Pain	Even More Pain	A Whole Lot Of Pain	Worst Pain

How was your energy today?
(mark with an X)

SPUNKY   DRAGGING

Notes:

_____

_____

_____

_____

_____

_____

TODAY'S DATE: _____

What was your body doing today?
(circle all that apply)

WORK

Sitting   Standing   Driving   Repetitive Movement

Speaking Gig   Phone Time   Computer Time

Other: _____

PLAY

Roughhousing with young kids   Tossing ball for the dog

Sitting on the floor

Other: _____

EXERCISE

Gym workout   Swim   Run   Yoga   Pilates

Bike (commute / stationary / trail)

Other: _____

Rate today's mood as well as your pain level:

Wong-Baker FACES® Pain Rating Scale

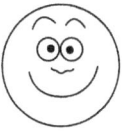 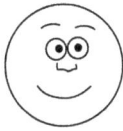 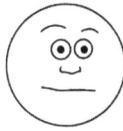 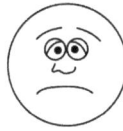 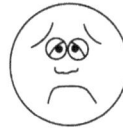 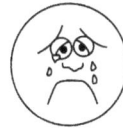

0	2	4	6	8	10
No Pain	A Little Pain	A Little More Pain	Even More Pain	A Whole Lot Of Pain	Worst Pain

How was your energy today?
(mark with an X)

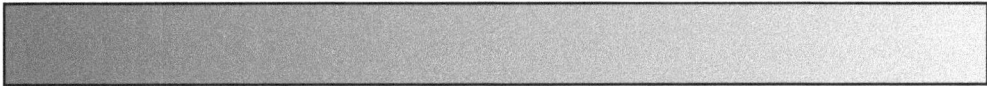

SPUNKY   DRAGGING

Notes:

_____

_____

_____

_____

_____

_____

_____

TODAY'S DATE: _____

What was your body doing today?
(circle all that apply)

WORK

Sitting   Standing   Driving   Repetitive Movement

Speaking Gig   Phone Time   Computer Time

Other: _____

PLAY

Roughhousing with young kids   Tossing ball for the dog

Sitting on the floor

Other: _____

EXERCISE

Gym workout   Swim   Run   Yoga   Pilates

Bike (commute / stationary / trail)

Other: _____

Rate today's mood as well as your pain level:

Wong-Baker FACES® Pain Rating Scale

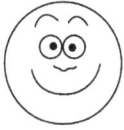 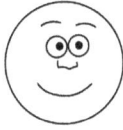 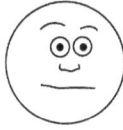 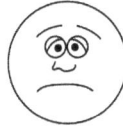 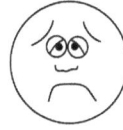 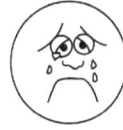

0	2	4	6	8	10
No Pain	A Little Pain	A Little More Pain	Even More Pain	A Whole Lot Of Pain	Worst Pain

How was your energy today?
(mark with an X)

SPUNKY   DRAGGING

Notes:

_____

_____

_____

_____

_____

_____

_____

TODAY'S DATE: _____

What was your body doing today?
(circle all that apply)

WORK

Sitting   Standing   Driving   Repetitive Movement

Speaking Gig   Phone Time   Computer Time

Other: _____

PLAY

Roughhousing with young kids   Tossing ball for the dog

Sitting on the floor

Other: _____

EXERCISE

Gym workout   Swim   Run   Yoga   Pilates

Bike (commute / stationary / trail)

Other: _____

Rate today's mood as well as your pain level:

Wong-Baker FACES® Pain Rating Scale

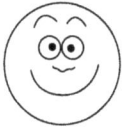 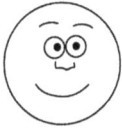 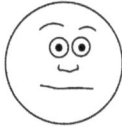 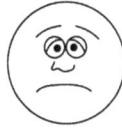 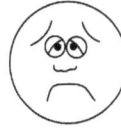 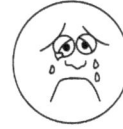

0	2	4	6	8	10
No Pain	A Little Pain	A Little More Pain	Even More Pain	A Whole Lot Of Pain	Worst Pain

How was your energy today?
(mark with an X)

SPUNKY   DRAGGING

Notes:

_____

_____

_____

_____

_____

_____

_____

YOU MADE IT TO THE END OF WEEK 4!

How are you feeling?

TODAY'S DATE: _____

PAIN LOCATION:
(circle one)

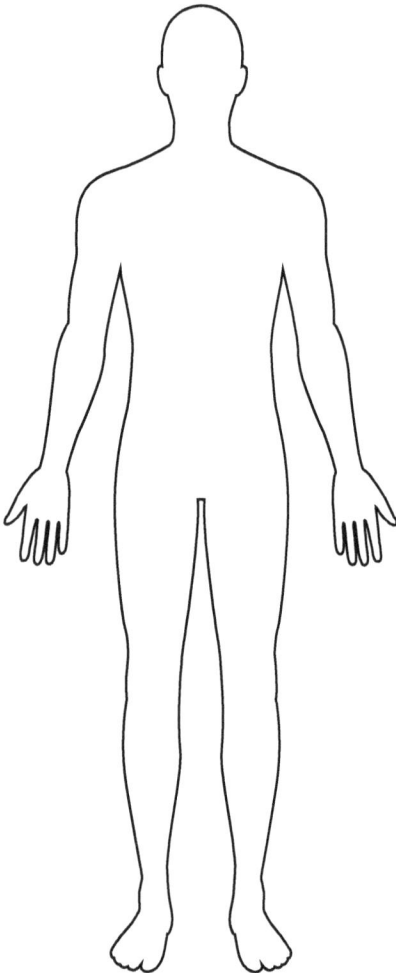

Neck

Neck/Shoulder

Shoulder/Upper Back

Mid Back/Torso/Ribs

Low Back

Low Back/Hip

Hip/Buttock/Thigh

*Use this figure to color or shade-in the area
of your pain however you like.*

HOW MUCH PAIN TODAY?

Circle the face below that best expresses your discomfort:

Wong-Baker FACES® Pain Rating Scale

0	2	4	6	8	10
No Pain	A Little Pain	A Little More Pain	Even More Pain	A Whole Lot Of Pain	Worst Pain

Notes:

_____

_____

_____

_____

_____

_____

_____

_____

_____

Digestion:
(circle all that apply)

Burping   Bloating   Passing gas   Belly pain

Constipation   Diarrhea/Loose stool

Other/More Details: _____

_____

_____

_____

_____

Breathing:
(circle all that apply)

Sniffly nose   Postnasal drip   Sinus congestion

Wheezing   Cough

Other/More Details: _____

_____

_____

_____

_____

Headaches:
(circle all that apply)

Forehead   Whole head   Right side   Left side

Other/More Details: _____

_____

_____

_____

_____

_____

Medication used:
(circle all that apply)

Inhaler   Antacids   Allergy tablets   Nasal spray/rinse

Ibuprofen (Motrin/Advil)   Naproxen (Aleve)

Aspirin   Acetaminophen (Tylenol)

Other/Prescription: _____

_____

How much? _____

_____

☐ Some Relief?   ☐ Total Relief?   ☐ No Relief?

REFLECTIONS

What worked? / What didn't work? Think about next steps: continue or try pausing one of the other Big Three triggers...

_____

_____

_____

_____

_____

_____

_____

_____

_____

_____

_____

_____

_____

AFFIRMATION:

Repeat out loud:

"My body chemistry is working hard to keep me safe, and I support it."

RELEASE THE SNEAKY THREE

Pick one or two of the sneaky **food sensitivities** and pause your intake for 3-5 days while playing with substitutions.

- At the end of 3-5 days, how do you feel? Are the substitutions working for you or are you thinking of trying different substitutions?
- You may not yet feel a difference in your body discomfort, but how is your belly feeling? Is your food going in and coming out comfortably? Are there other symptoms that have changed?

Consider where in your life you might experience exposure to any of the chemicals on the sneaky **chemical sensitivities** list.

- For storage of warm or acidic foods, use glass or metal containers instead of plastic.
- Try unscented and natural body and beauty products as well as laundry soap, dish detergents, and fabric softeners.
- Be careful with cleaning products, and always crack open a window in the vicinity when possible.
- Explore air purifiers, humidifiers, and/or dehumidifiers depending on the climate where you live.

Ask yourself if there is a **seasonal pattern** to your pain flare ups, especially if you also have a history of seasonal allergies. If so, investigate further how else to decrease your overall body burden since controlling exposure to pollen is less straightforward.

- Pay better attention to caring for your home environment to keep pollen at bay during those few months of the year that are the most challenging for you.
- Redirect your focus to modifying your exposure to the other sneaky three triggers or the big three during those vulnerable times of the year.

RELEASE - WEEK 1

START DATE: _____

Check one to three of the following things that you will pause or manage mindfully for the next 5-7 days.

Food Sensitivities to Release	Chemical Sensitivities to Release	Environmental Allergies to Release
☐ Dairy	☐ Petroleum	☐ Pollen
☐ Wheat	☐ PFAS	☐ Pet dander
☐ Caffeine	☐ Fragrances	☐ Dust mites
☐ Amines	☐ Cleaning products	☐ Mold
☐ Soy	☐ Diesel Fumes	
☐ Yeast	☐ Formaldehyde	
☐ Sulfites	☐ Epoxy	
☐ Salicylates	☐ Wildfire smoke	
☐ FODMAPs	You may not be able to avoid these, so just acknowledge and keep track of which environmental allergies your body is managing.	

Refer to *Fix the Fire Damage* for ideas about action steps to try and coping strategies. Jot them down here:

_____

_____

_____

TODAY'S DATE: _____

What was your body doing today?
(circle all that apply)

WORK

Sitting   Standing   Driving   Repetitive Movement

Speaking Gig   Phone Time   Computer Time

Other: _____

PLAY

Roughhousing with young kids   Tossing ball for the dog

Sitting on the floor

Other: _____

EXERCISE

Gym workout   Swim   Run   Yoga   Pilates

Bike (commute / stationary / trail)

Other: _____

Rate today's mood as well as your pain level:

Wong-Baker FACES® Pain Rating Scale

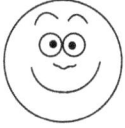 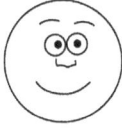 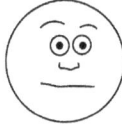 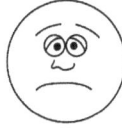 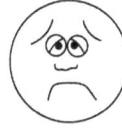 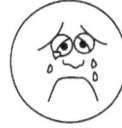

0	**2**	**4**	**6**	**8**	**10**
No Pain	A Little Pain	A Little More Pain	Even More Pain	A Whole Lot Of Pain	Worst Pain

How was your energy today?
(mark with an X)

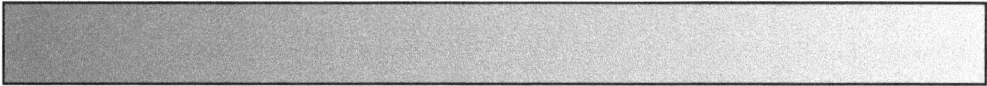

SPUNKY   DRAGGING

Notes:

_____

_____

_____

_____

_____

_____

_____

TODAY'S DATE: _____

What was your body doing today?
(circle all that apply)

WORK

Sitting   Standing   Driving   Repetitive Movement

Speaking Gig   Phone Time   Computer Time

Other: _____

PLAY

Roughhousing with young kids   Tossing ball for the dog

Sitting on the floor

Other: _____

EXERCISE

Gym workout   Swim   Run   Yoga   Pilates

Bike (commute / stationary / trail)

Other: _____

Rate today's mood as well as your pain level:

Wong-Baker FACES® Pain Rating Scale

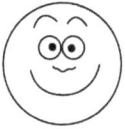 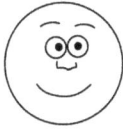 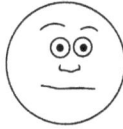 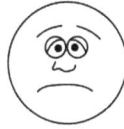 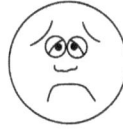 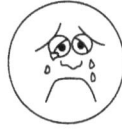

0	2	4	6	8	10
No Pain	A Little Pain	A Little More Pain	Even More Pain	A Whole Lot Of Pain	Worst Pain

How was your energy today?
(mark with an X)

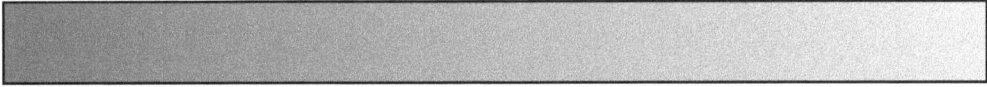

SPUNKY   DRAGGING

Notes:

_____

_____

_____

_____

_____

_____

_____

TODAY'S DATE: _____

What was your body doing today?
(circle all that apply)

WORK

Sitting   Standing   Driving   Repetitive Movement

Speaking Gig   Phone Time   Computer Time

Other: _____

PLAY

Roughhousing with young kids   Tossing ball for the dog

Sitting on the floor

Other: _____

EXERCISE

Gym workout   Swim   Run   Yoga   Pilates

Bike (commute / stationary / trail)

Other: _____

Rate today's mood as well as your pain level:

Wong-Baker FACES® Pain Rating Scale

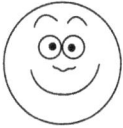 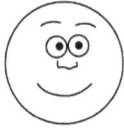 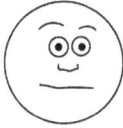 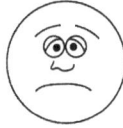 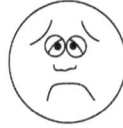 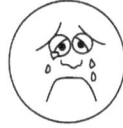

0	2	4	6	8	10
No Pain	A Little Pain	A Little More Pain	Even More Pain	A Whole Lot Of Pain	Worst Pain

How was your energy today?
(mark with an X)

SPUNKY   DRAGGING

Notes:

_____

_____

_____

_____

_____

_____

TODAY'S DATE: _____

What was your body doing today?
(circle all that apply)

WORK

Sitting   Standing   Driving   Repetitive Movement

Speaking Gig   Phone Time   Computer Time

Other: _____

PLAY

Roughhousing with young kids   Tossing ball for the dog

Sitting on the floor

Other: _____

EXERCISE

Gym workout   Swim   Run   Yoga   Pilates

Bike (commute / stationary / trail)

Other: _____

Rate today's mood as well as your pain level:

Wong-Baker FACES® Pain Rating Scale

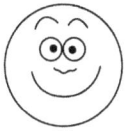 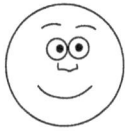 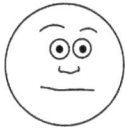 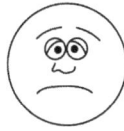 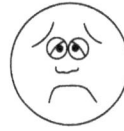 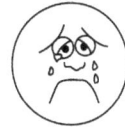

0	2	4	6	8	10
No Pain	A Little Pain	A Little More Pain	Even More Pain	A Whole Lot Of Pain	Worst Pain

How was your energy today?
(mark with an X)

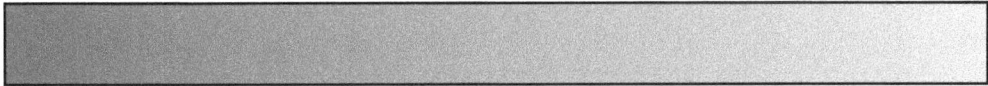

SPUNKY   DRAGGING

Notes:

_____

_____

_____

_____

_____

_____

TODAY'S DATE: _____

What was your body doing today?
(circle all that apply)

WORK

Sitting   Standing   Driving   Repetitive Movement

Speaking Gig   Phone Time   Computer Time

Other: _____

PLAY

Roughhousing with young kids   Tossing ball for the dog

Sitting on the floor

Other: _____

EXERCISE

Gym workout   Swim   Run   Yoga   Pilates

Bike (commute / stationary / trail)

Other: _____

Rate today's mood as well as your pain level:

Wong-Baker FACES® Pain Rating Scale

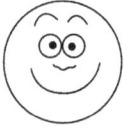 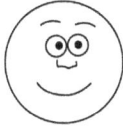 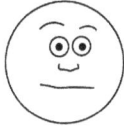 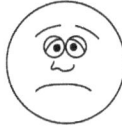 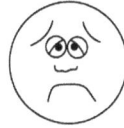 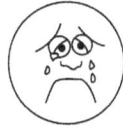

0	2	4	6	8	10
No Pain	A Little Pain	A Little More Pain	Even More Pain	A Whole Lot Of Pain	Worst Pain

How was your energy today?
(mark with an X)

SPUNKY   DRAGGING

Notes:

_____

_____

_____

_____

_____

_____

_____

TODAY'S DATE: _____

What was your body doing today?
(circle all that apply)

WORK

Sitting   Standing   Driving   Repetitive Movement

Speaking Gig   Phone Time   Computer Time

Other: _____

PLAY

Roughhousing with young kids   Tossing ball for the dog

Sitting on the floor

Other: _____

EXERCISE

Gym workout   Swim   Run   Yoga   Pilates

Bike (commute / stationary / trail)

Other: _____

Rate today's mood as well as your pain level:

Wong-Baker FACES® Pain Rating Scale

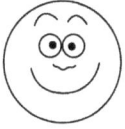 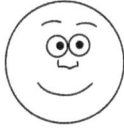 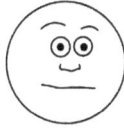 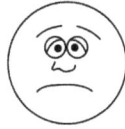 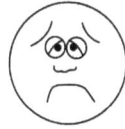 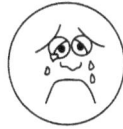

0	**2**	**4**	**6**	**8**	**10**
No Pain	A Little Pain	A Little More Pain	Even More Pain	A Whole Lot Of Pain	Worst Pain

How was your energy today?
(mark with an X)

SPUNKY   DRAGGING

Notes:

_____

_____

_____

_____

_____

_____

TODAY'S DATE: _____

What was your body doing today?
(circle all that apply)

WORK

Sitting   Standing   Driving   Repetitive Movement

Speaking Gig   Phone Time   Computer Time

Other: _____

PLAY

Roughhousing with young kids   Tossing ball for the dog

Sitting on the floor

Other: _____

EXERCISE

Gym workout   Swim   Run   Yoga   Pilates

Bike (commute / stationary / trail)

Other: _____

Rate today's mood as well as your pain level:

Wong-Baker FACES® Pain Rating Scale

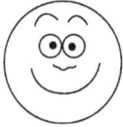 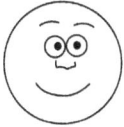 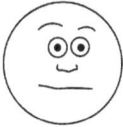 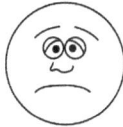 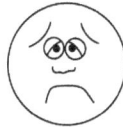 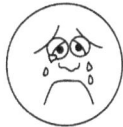

0	2	4	6	8	10
No Pain	A Little Pain	A Little More Pain	Even More Pain	A Whole Lot Of Pain	Worst Pain

How was your energy today?
(mark with an X)

SPUNKY   DRAGGING

Notes:

_____

_____

_____

_____

_____

_____

_____

AFFIRMATION:

Repeat out loud:

"I choose foods that calm my body and free me from pain."

RELEASE - WEEK 2

START DATE: _____

Check one to three of the following things that you will pause or manage mindfully for the next 5-7 days.

Food Sensitivities to Release	Chemical Sensitivities to Release	Environmental Allergies to Release
☐ Dairy	☐ Petroleum	☐ Pollen
☐ Wheat	☐ PFAS	☐ Pet dander
☐ Caffeine	☐ Fragrances	☐ Dust mites
☐ Amines	☐ Cleaning products	☐ Mold
☐ Soy	☐ Diesel Fumes	
☐ Yeast	☐ Formaldehyde	
☐ Sulfites	☐ Epoxy	
☐ Salicylates	☐ Wildfire smoke	
☐ FODMAPs	You may not be able to avoid these, so just acknowledge and keep track of which environmental allergies your body is managing.	

Refer to *Fix the Fire Damage* for ideas about action steps to try and coping strategies. Jot them down here:

_____

_____

_____

TODAY'S DATE: _____

What was your body doing today?
(circle all that apply)

WORK

Sitting   Standing   Driving   Repetitive Movement

Speaking Gig   Phone Time   Computer Time

Other: _____

PLAY

Roughhousing with young kids   Tossing ball for the dog

Sitting on the floor

Other: _____

EXERCISE

Gym workout   Swim   Run   Yoga   Pilates

Bike (commute / stationary / trail)

Other: _____

Rate today's mood as well as your pain level:

Wong-Baker FACES® Pain Rating Scale

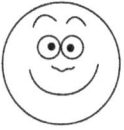 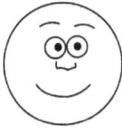 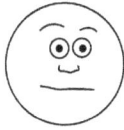 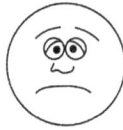 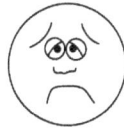 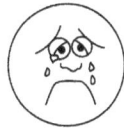

0	2	4	6	8	10
No Pain	A Little Pain	A Little More Pain	Even More Pain	A Whole Lot Of Pain	Worst Pain

How was your energy today?
(mark with an X)

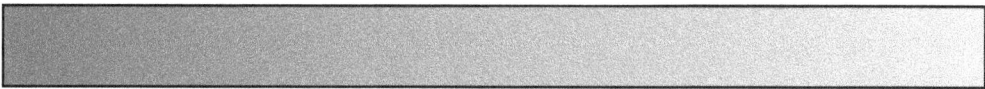

SPUNKY   DRAGGING

Notes:

_____

_____

_____

_____

_____

_____

_____

TODAY'S DATE: _____

What was your body doing today?
(circle all that apply)

WORK

Sitting   Standing   Driving   Repetitive Movement

Speaking Gig   Phone Time   Computer Time

Other: _____

PLAY

Roughhousing with young kids   Tossing ball for the dog

Sitting on the floor

Other: _____

EXERCISE

Gym workout   Swim   Run   Yoga   Pilates

Bike (commute / stationary / trail)

Other: _____

Rate today's mood as well as your pain level:

Wong-Baker FACES® Pain Rating Scale

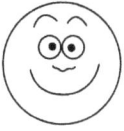 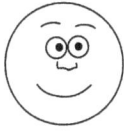 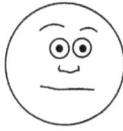 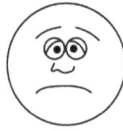 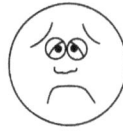 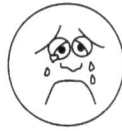

0	**2**	**4**	**6**	**8**	**10**
No Pain	A Little Pain	A Little More Pain	Even More Pain	A Whole Lot Of Pain	Worst Pain

How was your energy today?
(mark with an X)

SPUNKY   DRAGGING

Notes:

_____

_____

_____

_____

_____

_____

_____

TODAY'S DATE: _____

What was your body doing today?
(circle all that apply)

WORK

Sitting   Standing   Driving   Repetitive Movement

Speaking Gig   Phone Time   Computer Time

Other: _____

PLAY

Roughhousing with young kids   Tossing ball for the dog

Sitting on the floor

Other: _____

EXERCISE

Gym workout   Swim   Run   Yoga   Pilates

Bike (commute / stationary / trail)

Other: _____

Rate today's mood as well as your pain level:

Wong-Baker FACES® Pain Rating Scale

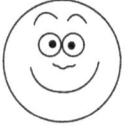 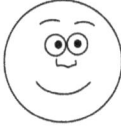 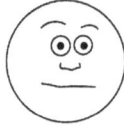 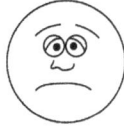 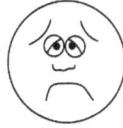 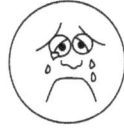

0	**2**	**4**	**6**	**8**	**10**
No Pain	A Little Pain	A Little More Pain	Even More Pain	A Whole Lot Of Pain	Worst Pain

How was your energy today?
(mark with an X)

SPUNKY   DRAGGING

Notes:

_____

_____

_____

_____

_____

_____

TODAY'S DATE: _____

What was your body doing today?
(circle all that apply)

WORK

Sitting   Standing   Driving   Repetitive Movement

Speaking Gig   Phone Time   Computer Time

Other: _____

PLAY

Roughhousing with young kids   Tossing ball for the dog

Sitting on the floor

Other: _____

EXERCISE

Gym workout   Swim   Run   Yoga   Pilates

Bike (commute / stationary / trail)

Other: _____

Rate today's mood as well as your pain level:

Wong-Baker FACES® Pain Rating Scale

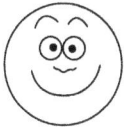 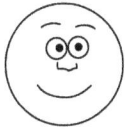 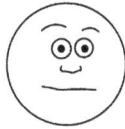 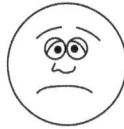 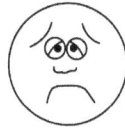 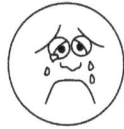

0	2	4	6	8	10
No Pain	A Little Pain	A Little More Pain	Even More Pain	A Whole Lot Of Pain	Worst Pain

How was your energy today?
(mark with an X)

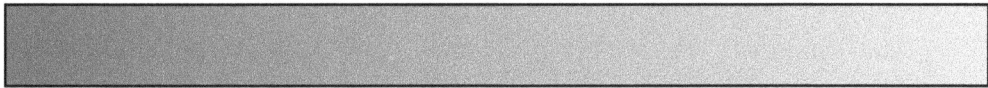

SPUNKY   DRAGGING

Notes:

_____

_____

_____

_____

_____

_____

TODAY'S DATE: _____

What was your body doing today?
(circle all that apply)

WORK

Sitting   Standing   Driving   Repetitive Movement

Speaking Gig   Phone Time   Computer Time

Other: _____

PLAY

Roughhousing with young kids   Tossing ball for the dog

Sitting on the floor

Other: _____

EXERCISE

Gym workout   Swim   Run   Yoga   Pilates

Bike (commute / stationary / trail)

Other: _____

Rate today's mood as well as your pain level:

Wong-Baker FACES® Pain Rating Scale

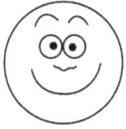 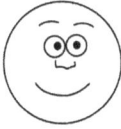 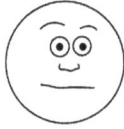 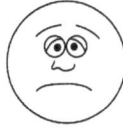 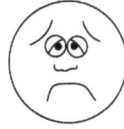 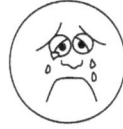

0	2	4	6	8	10
No Pain	A Little Pain	A Little More Pain	Even More Pain	A Whole Lot Of Pain	Worst Pain

How was your energy today?
(mark with an X)

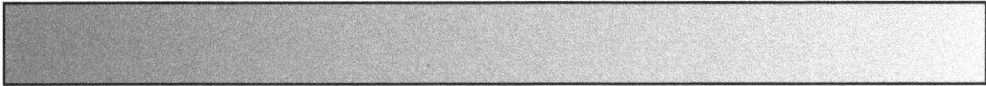

SPUNKY   DRAGGING

Notes:

_____

_____

_____

_____

_____

_____

TODAY'S DATE: _____

What was your body doing today?
(circle all that apply)

WORK

Sitting Standing Driving Repetitive Movement

Speaking Gig Phone Time Computer Time

Other: _____

PLAY

Roughhousing with young kids Tossing ball for the dog

Sitting on the floor

Other: _____

EXERCISE

Gym workout Swim Run Yoga Pilates

Bike (commute / stationary / trail)

Other: _____

Rate today's mood as well as your pain level:

Wong-Baker FACES® Pain Rating Scale

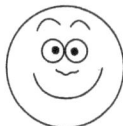 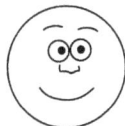 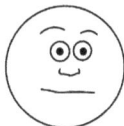 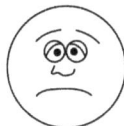 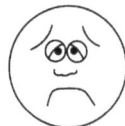 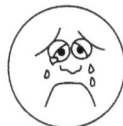

0	**2**	**4**	**6**	**8**	**10**
No Pain	A Little Pain	A Little More Pain	Even More Pain	A Whole Lot Of Pain	Worst Pain

How was your energy today?
(mark with an X)

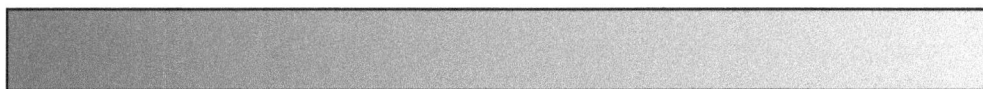

SPUNKY   DRAGGING

Notes:

_____

_____

_____

_____

_____

_____

_____

TODAY'S DATE: _____

What was your body doing today?
(circle all that apply)

WORK

Sitting   Standing   Driving   Repetitive Movement

Speaking Gig   Phone Time   Computer Time

Other: _____

PLAY

Roughhousing with young kids   Tossing ball for the dog

Sitting on the floor

Other: _____

EXERCISE

Gym workout   Swim   Run   Yoga   Pilates

Bike (commute / stationary / trail)

Other: _____

Rate today's mood as well as your pain level:

Wong-Baker FACES® Pain Rating Scale

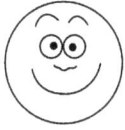 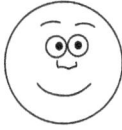 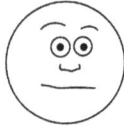 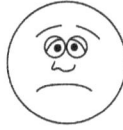 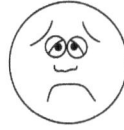 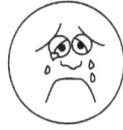

0	2	4	6	8	10
No Pain	A Little Pain	A Little More Pain	Even More Pain	A Whole Lot Of Pain	Worst Pain

How was your energy today?
(mark with an X)

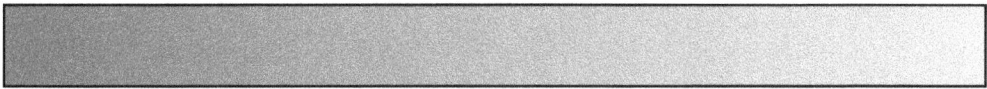

SPUNKY   DRAGGING

Notes:

_____

_____

_____

_____

_____

_____

_____

AFFIRMATION:

Repeat out loud:

"With every clean choice, I unburden my body and allow myself to heal more quickly."

RELEASE – WEEK 3

START DATE: _____

Check one to three of the following things that you will pause or manage mindfully for the next 5-7 days.

Food Sensitivities to Release	Chemical Sensitivities to Release	Environmental Allergies to Release
☐ Dairy	☐ Petroleum	☐ Pollen
☐ Wheat	☐ PFAS	☐ Pet dander
☐ Caffeine	☐ Fragrances	☐ Dust mites
☐ Amines	☐ Cleaning products	☐ Mold
☐ Soy	☐ Diesel Fumes	
☐ Yeast	☐ Formaldehyde	
☐ Sulfites	☐ Epoxy	
☐ Salicylates	☐ Wildfire smoke	
☐ FODMAPs	You may not be able to avoid these, so just acknowledge and keep track of which environmental allergies your body is managing.	

Refer to *Fix the Fire Damage* for ideas about action steps to try and coping strategies. Jot them down here:

_____

_____

_____

TODAY'S DATE: _____

What was your body doing today?
(circle all that apply)

WORK

Sitting   Standing   Driving   Repetitive Movement

Speaking Gig   Phone Time   Computer Time

Other: _____

PLAY

Roughhousing with young kids   Tossing ball for the dog

Sitting on the floor

Other: _____

EXERCISE

Gym workout   Swim   Run   Yoga   Pilates

Bike (commute / stationary / trail)

Other: _____

Rate today's mood as well as your pain level:

Wong-Baker FACES® Pain Rating Scale

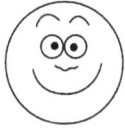 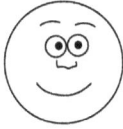 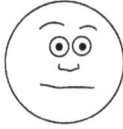 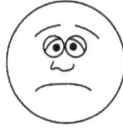 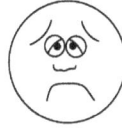 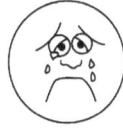

0	**2**	**4**	**6**	**8**	**10**
No Pain	A Little Pain	A Little More Pain	Even More Pain	A Whole Lot Of Pain	Worst Pain

How was your energy today?
(mark with an X)

SPUNKY   DRAGGING

Notes:

_____

_____

_____

_____

_____

_____

TODAY'S DATE: _____

What was your body doing today?
(circle all that apply)

WORK

Sitting   Standing   Driving   Repetitive Movement

Speaking Gig   Phone Time   Computer Time

Other: _____

PLAY

Roughhousing with young kids   Tossing ball for the dog

Sitting on the floor

Other: _____

EXERCISE

Gym workout   Swim   Run   Yoga   Pilates

Bike (commute / stationary / trail)

Other: _____

Rate today's mood as well as your pain level:

Wong-Baker FACES® Pain Rating Scale

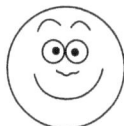 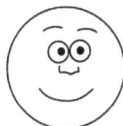 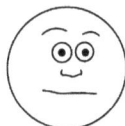 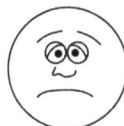 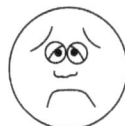 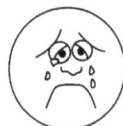

0	**2**	**4**	**6**	**8**	**10**
No Pain	A Little Pain	A Little More Pain	Even More Pain	A Whole Lot Of Pain	Worst Pain

How was your energy today?
(mark with an X)

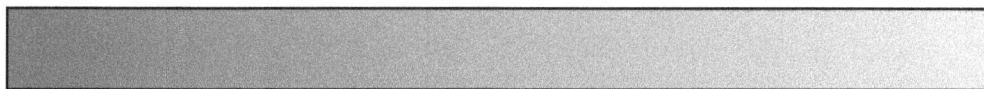

SPUNKY   DRAGGING

Notes:

_____

_____

_____

_____

_____

_____

RELEASE – WEEK 3

TODAY'S DATE: _____

What was your body doing today?
(circle all that apply)

WORK

Sitting   Standing   Driving   Repetitive Movement

Speaking Gig   Phone Time   Computer Time

Other: _____

PLAY

Roughhousing with young kids   Tossing ball for the dog

Sitting on the floor

Other: _____

EXERCISE

Gym workout   Swim   Run   Yoga   Pilates

Bike (commute / stationary / trail)

Other: _____

Rate today's mood as well as your pain level:

Wong-Baker FACES® Pain Rating Scale

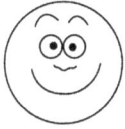 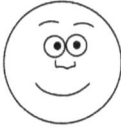 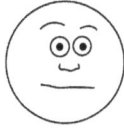 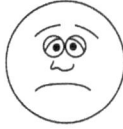 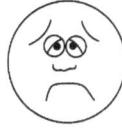 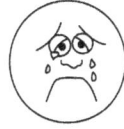

0	2	4	6	8	10
No Pain	A Little Pain	A Little More Pain	Even More Pain	A Whole Lot Of Pain	Worst Pain

How was your energy today?
(mark with an X)

SPUNKY   DRAGGING

Notes:

_____

_____

_____

_____

_____

_____

TODAY'S DATE: _____

What was your body doing today?
(circle all that apply)

WORK

Sitting   Standing   Driving   Repetitive Movement

Speaking Gig   Phone Time   Computer Time

Other: _____

PLAY

Roughhousing with young kids   Tossing ball for the dog

Sitting on the floor

Other: _____

EXERCISE

Gym workout   Swim   Run   Yoga   Pilates

Bike (commute / stationary / trail)

Other: _____

Rate today's mood as well as your pain level:

Wong-Baker FACES® Pain Rating Scale

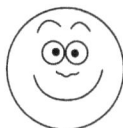 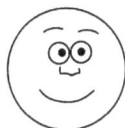 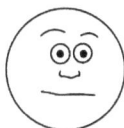 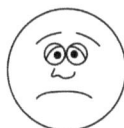 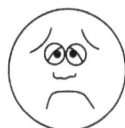 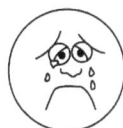

0	**2**	**4**	**6**	**8**	**10**
No Pain	A Little Pain	A Little More Pain	Even More Pain	A Whole Lot Of Pain	Worst Pain

How was your energy today?
(mark with an X)

SPUNKY   DRAGGING

Notes:

_____

_____

_____

_____

_____

_____

TODAY'S DATE: _____

What was your body doing today?
(circle all that apply)

WORK

Sitting   Standing   Driving   Repetitive Movement

Speaking Gig   Phone Time   Computer Time

Other: _____

PLAY

Roughhousing with young kids   Tossing ball for the dog

Sitting on the floor

Other: _____

EXERCISE

Gym workout   Swim   Run   Yoga   Pilates

Bike (commute / stationary / trail)

Other: _____

Rate today's mood as well as your pain level:

Wong-Baker FACES® Pain Rating Scale

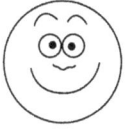 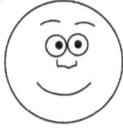 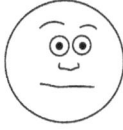 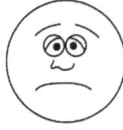 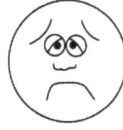 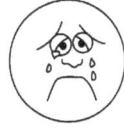

0	2	4	6	8	10
No Pain	A Little Pain	A Little More Pain	Even More Pain	A Whole Lot Of Pain	Worst Pain

How was your energy today?
(mark with an X)

SPUNKY   DRAGGING

Notes:

_____

_____

_____

_____

_____

_____

_____

TODAY'S DATE: _____

What was your body doing today?
(circle all that apply)

WORK

Sitting   Standing   Driving   Repetitive Movement

Speaking Gig   Phone Time   Computer Time

Other: _____

PLAY

Roughhousing with young kids   Tossing ball for the dog

Sitting on the floor

Other: _____

EXERCISE

Gym workout   Swim   Run   Yoga   Pilates

Bike (commute / stationary / trail)

Other: _____

Rate today's mood as well as your pain level:

Wong-Baker FACES® Pain Rating Scale

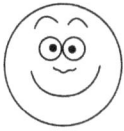 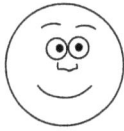 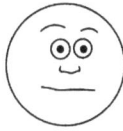 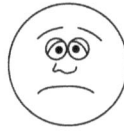 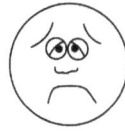 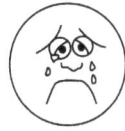

0	2	4	6	8	10
No Pain	A Little Pain	A Little More Pain	Even More Pain	A Whole Lot Of Pain	Worst Pain

How was your energy today?
(mark with an X)

SPUNKY   DRAGGING

Notes:

_____

_____

_____

_____

_____

_____

TODAY'S DATE: _____

What was your body doing today?
(circle all that apply)

WORK

Sitting   Standing   Driving   Repetitive Movement

Speaking Gig   Phone Time   Computer Time

Other: _____

PLAY

Roughhousing with young kids   Tossing ball for the dog

Sitting on the floor

Other: _____

EXERCISE

Gym workout   Swim   Run   Yoga   Pilates

Bike (commute / stationary / trail)

Other: _____

Rate today's mood as well as your pain level:

Wong-Baker FACES® Pain Rating Scale

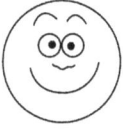 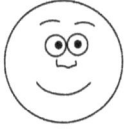 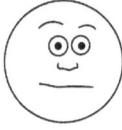 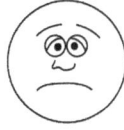 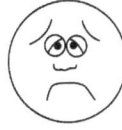 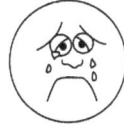

0	2	4	6	8	10
No Pain	A Little Pain	A Little More Pain	Even More Pain	A Whole Lot Of Pain	Worst Pain

How was your energy today?
(mark with an X)

SPUNKY   DRAGGING

Notes:

_____

_____

_____

_____

_____

_____

AFFIRMATION:

Repeat out loud:

"With each day, my body chemistry is returning to its naturally wise and effortless state: powerful, precise and unstoppable."

RELEASE - WEEK 4

START DATE: _____

Check one to three of the following things that you will pause or manage mindfully for the next 5-7 days.

Food Sensitivities to Release	Chemical Sensitivities to Release	Environmental Allergies to Release
☐ Dairy	☐ Petroleum	☐ Pollen
☐ Wheat	☐ PFAS	☐ Pet dander
☐ Caffeine	☐ Fragrances	☐ Dust mites
☐ Amines	☐ Cleaning products	☐ Mold
☐ Soy	☐ Diesel Fumes	
☐ Yeast	☐ Formaldehyde	
☐ Sulfites	☐ Epoxy	
☐ Salicylates	☐ Wildfire smoke	
☐ FODMAPs	You may not be able to avoid these, so just acknowledge and keep track of which environmental allergies your body is managing.	

Refer to *Fix the Fire Damage* for ideas about action steps to try and coping strategies. Jot them down here:

_____

_____

_____

RELEASE – WEEK 4

TODAY'S DATE: _____

What was your body doing today?
(circle all that apply)

WORK

Sitting   Standing   Driving   Repetitive Movement

Speaking Gig   Phone Time   Computer Time

Other: _____

PLAY

Roughhousing with young kids   Tossing ball for the dog

Sitting on the floor

Other: _____

EXERCISE

Gym workout   Swim   Run   Yoga   Pilates

Bike (commute / stationary / trail)

Other: _____

Rate today's mood as well as your pain level:

Wong-Baker FACES® Pain Rating Scale

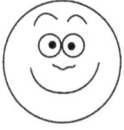 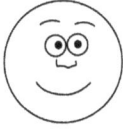 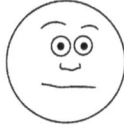 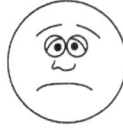 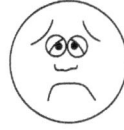 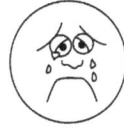

0	**2**	**4**	**6**	**8**	**10**
No Pain	A Little Pain	A Little More Pain	Even More Pain	A Whole Lot Of Pain	Worst Pain

How was your energy today?
(mark with an X)

SPUNKY   DRAGGING

Notes:

_____

_____

_____

_____

_____

_____

_____

TODAY'S DATE: _____

What was your body doing today?
(circle all that apply)

WORK

Sitting   Standing   Driving   Repetitive Movement

Speaking Gig   Phone Time   Computer Time

Other: _____

PLAY

Roughhousing with young kids   Tossing ball for the dog

Sitting on the floor

Other: _____

EXERCISE

Gym workout   Swim   Run   Yoga   Pilates

Bike (commute / stationary / trail)

Other: _____

Rate today's mood as well as your pain level:

Wong-Baker FACES® Pain Rating Scale

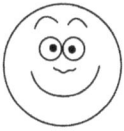 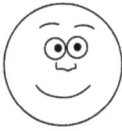 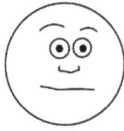 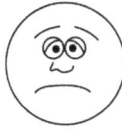 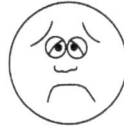 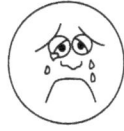

0	**2**	**4**	**6**	**8**	**10**
No Pain	A Little Pain	A Little More Pain	Even More Pain	A Whole Lot Of Pain	Worst Pain

How was your energy today?
(mark with an X)

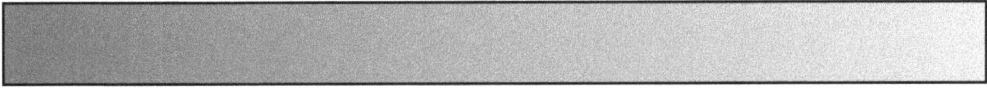

SPUNKY   DRAGGING

Notes:

_____

_____

_____

_____

_____

_____

TODAY'S DATE: _____

What was your body doing today?
(circle all that apply)

WORK

Sitting   Standing   Driving   Repetitive Movement

Speaking Gig   Phone Time   Computer Time

Other: _____

PLAY

Roughhousing with young kids   Tossing ball for the dog

Sitting on the floor

Other: _____

EXERCISE

Gym workout   Swim   Run   Yoga   Pilates

Bike (commute / stationary / trail)

Other: _____

Rate today's mood as well as your pain level:

Wong-Baker FACES® Pain Rating Scale

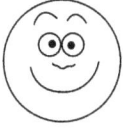 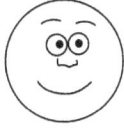 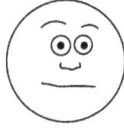 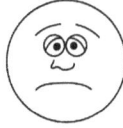 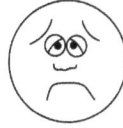 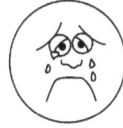

0	2	4	6	8	10
No Pain	A Little Pain	A Little More Pain	Even More Pain	A Whole Lot Of Pain	Worst Pain

How was your energy today?
(mark with an X)

SPUNKY   DRAGGING

Notes:

_____

_____

_____

_____

_____

_____

TODAY'S DATE: _____

What was your body doing today?
(circle all that apply)

WORK

Sitting   Standing   Driving   Repetitive Movement

Speaking Gig   Phone Time   Computer Time

Other: _____

PLAY

Roughhousing with young kids   Tossing ball for the dog

Sitting on the floor

Other: _____

EXERCISE

Gym workout   Swim   Run   Yoga   Pilates

Bike (commute / stationary / trail)

Other: _____

Rate today's mood as well as your pain level:

Wong-Baker FACES® Pain Rating Scale

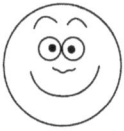 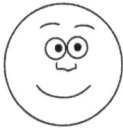 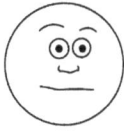 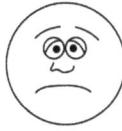 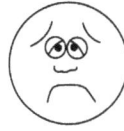 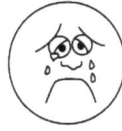

0	2	4	6	8	10
No Pain	A Little Pain	A Little More Pain	Even More Pain	A Whole Lot Of Pain	Worst Pain

How was your energy today?
(mark with an X)

SPUNKY   DRAGGING

Notes:

_____

_____

_____

_____

_____

_____

TODAY'S DATE: _____

What was your body doing today?
(circle all that apply)

WORK

     Sitting   Standing   Driving   Repetitive Movement

     Speaking Gig   Phone Time   Computer Time

Other: _____

PLAY

     Roughhousing with young kids   Tossing ball for the dog

     Sitting on the floor

Other: _____

EXERCISE

     Gym workout   Swim   Run   Yoga   Pilates

     Bike (commute / stationary / trail)

Other: _____

Rate today's mood as well as your pain level:

Wong-Baker FACES® Pain Rating Scale

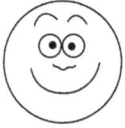 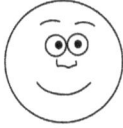 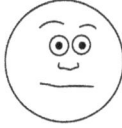 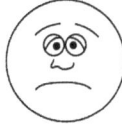 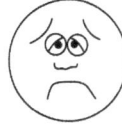 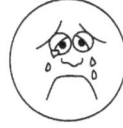

0	**2**	**4**	**6**	**8**	**10**
No Pain	A Little Pain	A Little More Pain	Even More Pain	A Whole Lot Of Pain	Worst Pain

How was your energy today?
(mark with an X)

SPUNKY   DRAGGING

Notes:

_____

_____

_____

_____

_____

_____

TODAY'S DATE: _____

What was your body doing today?
(circle all that apply)

WORK

Sitting   Standing   Driving   Repetitive Movement

Speaking Gig   Phone Time   Computer Time

Other: _____

PLAY

Roughhousing with young kids   Tossing ball for the dog

Sitting on the floor

Other: _____

EXERCISE

Gym workout   Swim   Run   Yoga   Pilates

Bike (commute / stationary / trail)

Other: _____

Rate today's mood as well as your pain level:

Wong-Baker FACES® Pain Rating Scale

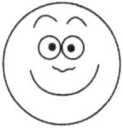 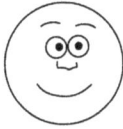 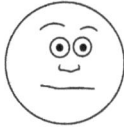 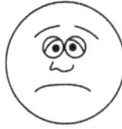 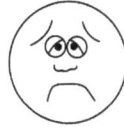 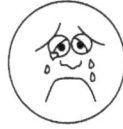

0	**2**	**4**	**6**	**8**	**10**
No Pain	A Little Pain	A Little More Pain	Even More Pain	A Whole Lot Of Pain	Worst Pain

How was your energy today?
(mark with an X)

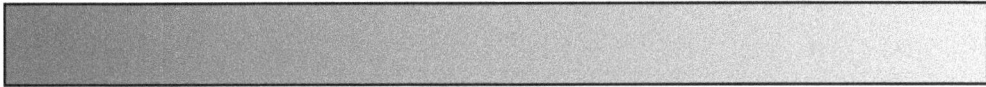

SPUNKY   DRAGGING

Notes:

_____

_____

_____

_____

_____

_____

TODAY'S DATE: _____

What was your body doing today?
(circle all that apply)

WORK

Sitting   Standing   Driving   Repetitive Movement

Speaking Gig   Phone Time   Computer Time

Other: _____

PLAY

Roughhousing with young kids   Tossing ball for the dog

Sitting on the floor

Other: _____

EXERCISE

Gym workout   Swim   Run   Yoga   Pilates

Bike (commute / stationary / trail)

Other: _____

Rate today's mood as well as your pain level:

Wong-Baker FACES® Pain Rating Scale

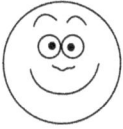 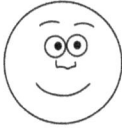 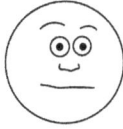 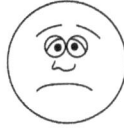 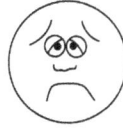 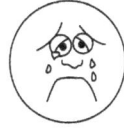

0	**2**	**4**	**6**	**8**	**10**
No Pain	A Little Pain	A Little More Pain	Even More Pain	A Whole Lot Of Pain	Worst Pain

How was your energy today?
(mark with an X)

SPUNKY   DRAGGING

Notes:

_____

_____

_____

_____

_____

_____

RELEASE

Are you ready for the next phase of action - Retrain?

Q: Do you still have some of the following:

- Minor but ongoing neck, shoulder, back, or hip pain
- Minor digestive discomfort(bloating, heartburn, constipation, or loose stool)
- Headaches
- Minor upper respiratory symptoms (including postnasal drip)
- Skin rashes
- Other_____

Details:_____

_____

_____

_____

_____

_____

_____

_____

_____

Q: Have you explored spending one to two weeks in the Release phase by taking a break from at least one of the big three burdensome garbage items?

Circle one: Yes / No

Details: _____

_____

_____

_____

_____

_____

_____

If you answered YES to any of the above, then you are ready to try the Retrain activities.

There is no wrong time to implement the Retrain phase of the Body Chemistry Action Plan. You can use these strategies simultaneously with Action Phase 1: Release. Just keep in mind that doing one thing at a time can give you better information about what's actually working, and it's often less overwhelming to change one thing at a time.

My *Retrain* Action Steps

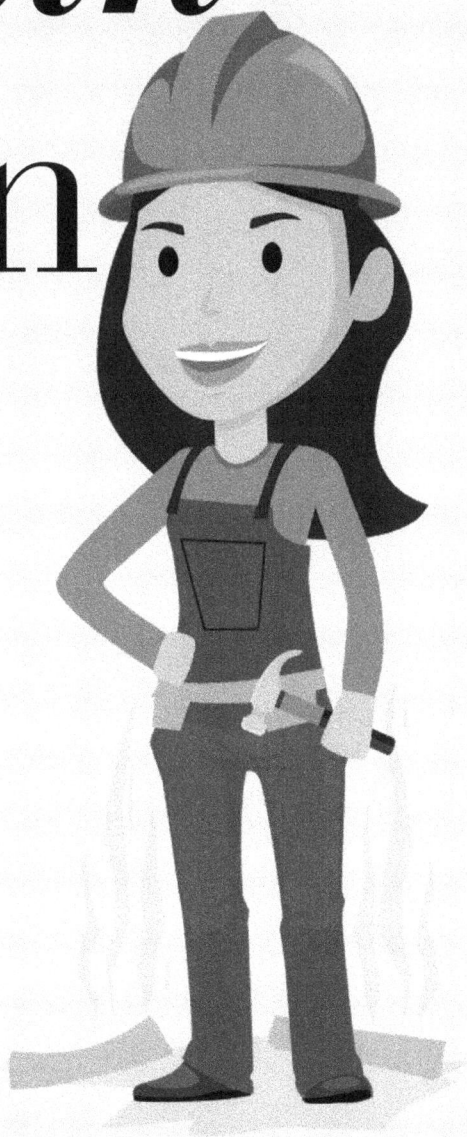

RETRAIN!

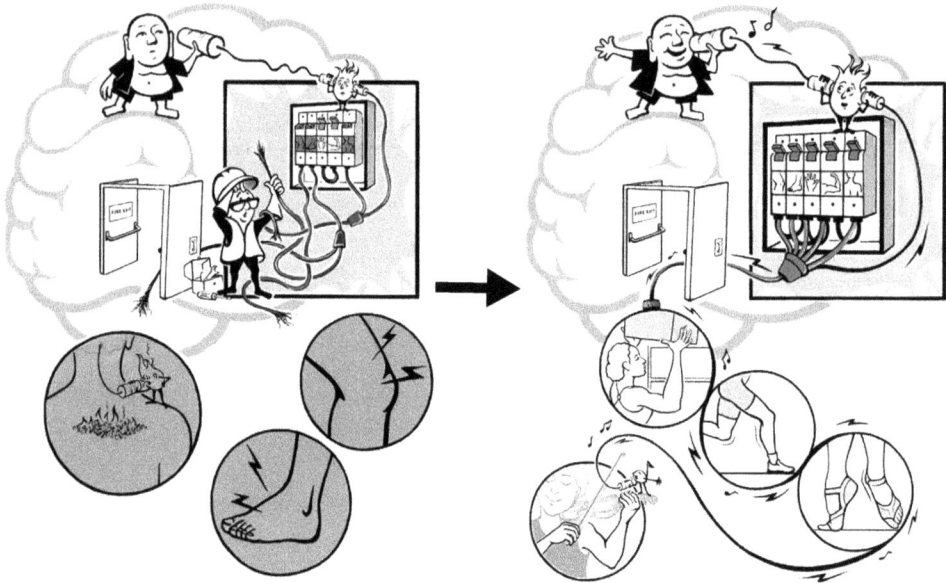

Q: *What* are you retraining?

A: **Your three garbage journeys to each run more smoothly**

Q: *How* are you retraining your garbage journeys?

A: **By helping or getting out of the way of your garbage influencers**

➤ Go to the book for more: *Fix the Fire Damage*, pages 427 – 440

➤ Listen to the podcast: *Conversations About Everyday Pain*, Season 2, Episodes 36 - 39

NEXT STEPS:

1. Support your garbage influencers

2. Support your liver auto-detox steps 1 and 2

3. Support the repair and maintenance of your gut wall

SUPPORT YOUR GARBAGE INFLUENCERS

Garbage Influencers	Ways to Support	Obstacles to Remove
Teeth		
Saliva		
Pancreas		
Gallbladder		

Need ideas? Refer to *Fix the Fire Damage* page 428 – 432.

Garbage Influencers	Ways to Support	Obstacles to Remove
Mucus membranes		
Hair cells		
Immune cells		
Epidermis		

My
Garbage
Influencers
Journal

_____

_____

_____

_____

_____

_____

_____

_____

_____

_____

_____

_____

_____

_____

_____

_____

_____

_____

_____

_____

_____

_____

_____

_____

_____

_____

_____

_____

_____

_____

_____

_____

MY GARBAGE INFLUENCERS JOURNAL

SUPPORT YOUR LIVER AUTO-DETOX

Liver auto-detox step 1 – specialized enzyme support:

Check one or more of the following can you add or increase in your daily food intake?

- ☐ Cruciferous vegetables (broccoli/cauliflower/brussels sprouts etc.)
- ☐ Curcumin
- ☐ Garlic
- ☐ Fish oil
- ☐ Rosemary
- ☐ Green tea
- ☐ Black tea

Liver auto-detox step 2 – neutralizer molecule support:

Check and circle any of the following that you agree to add or increase in your daily food intake:

- ☐ Dark green leafy vegetables
- ☐ Spinach, beets, whole grains, and crustaceans
- ☐ Meat, fish, poultry, dairy, and eggs
- ☐ Eggs, fish, and some meats
- ☐ Dairy, eggs, organ meats,
- ☐ Nutritional yeast, and seaweed
- ☐ Pumpkin seeds, almonds, and spinach
- ☐ Shellfish like oysters, meat, legumes, and seeds
- ☐ Legumes (in particular), whole grains, nuts, and beef liver

Refer to *Fix the Fire Damage* page 434 – 435.

My Liver Auto-Detox Journal

_____

_____

_____

_____

_____

_____

_____

_____

_____

_____

_____

_____

_____

_____

_____

_____

_____

_____

MY LIVER AUTO-DETOX JOURNAL

_____

_____

_____

_____

_____

_____

_____

_____

_____

_____

_____

_____

_____

_____

_____

_____

_____

_____

_____

_____

_____

_____

_____

_____

_____

_____

_____

_____

_____

_____

_____

_____

_____

SUPPORT YOUR
GUT WALL

Support a healthy gut wall by plugging the leaks!

Check and circle any of the following to increase in your daily food intake for less gut permeability:

- [ ] **Foods high in fiber** like legumes, beans, and oats.

- [ ] **Vitamin D** from sun exposure, or eating mushrooms, fatty fish, egg yolks and cod liver oil.

- [ ] **Vitamin A** found in dark green leafy vegetables, red or orange foods grown in the garden, and organ meats like liver.

- [ ] **Zinc** is found in whole grains, some seafood, legumes, meat, and poultry.

- [ ] **Anthocyanins** colored pigments found in red to purplish-blue foods like berries, leafy vegetables, roots, and tubers.

- [ ] **Cysteine** from foods like pork, beef, chicken, fish, lentils, oatmeal, eggs, low-fat yogurt, sunflower seeds, and cheese.

- [ ] **Methionine** from turkey, beef, fish, pork, tofu, milk, cheese, nuts, beans, and whole grains like quinoa.

- [ ] **Glutamine** from uncooked foods like raw cabbage (and red cabbage in particular), raw beets, spinach, and parsley.

- [ ] **Tryptophan** is found in chicken, turkey, red meat, pork, tofu, fish, beans, milk, nuts, seeds, oatmeal, eggs, cheese, and chocolate.

- [ ] **Arginine** from nuts and seeds, meat products, legumes, and seaweed.

Check any of the following that you can commit to avoiding or decreasing for less gut permeability:

- [ ] **Gluten** is found in wheat products, which are included in the big three. Gluten is also a known sneaky three irritant.

- [ ] **Glucose** is the main sugar to avoid as part of the big three.

- [ ] **Fructose** is another sugar to avoid as part of the big three.

- [ ] **Fat**, particularly saturated fat, is something you're already limiting as part of the big three.

- [ ] **Ethanol** is the intoxicating molecule in alcohol that you're already avoiding as part of the big three.

- [ ] **Emulsifiers** are FDA-approved additives in processed/packaged food to keep ingredients like oil and water from separating. These are also already part of the big three.

Refer to *Fix the Fire Damage* page 434 – 435.

My
Gut
Health
Journal

_____

_____

_____

_____

_____

_____

_____

_____

_____

_____

_____

_____

_____

_____

_____

MY GUT HEALTH JOURNAL

Are you ready for the next phase of action - Reinforce?

Q: Have you discovered some of your unique garbage burdens through the Release process, and have you been able to take breaks from them here and there?

Circle one: Yes / No

Details:_____

_____

_____

_____

_____

Q: Have you spent some time learning how to assist your garbage influencers in the Retrain phase?

Circle one: Yes / No

Details:_____

_____

_____

_____

_____

Q: Do you feel overwhelmed by the Release and Retrain phases? It's okay to just start here.

Circle one: Yes / No

Details:_____

_____

_____

_____

_____

_____

If you answered YES to any of the above questions, then you are ready to try the Reinforce activities.

Body Chemistry Reinforce techniques will help you create an easier, unobstructed passage of burdensome garbage through each body-machine garbage journey. Keeping the garbage flowing instead of stagnating can help you to prevent future flare-ups and to become inflammation fireproof.

My *Reinforce* Action Steps

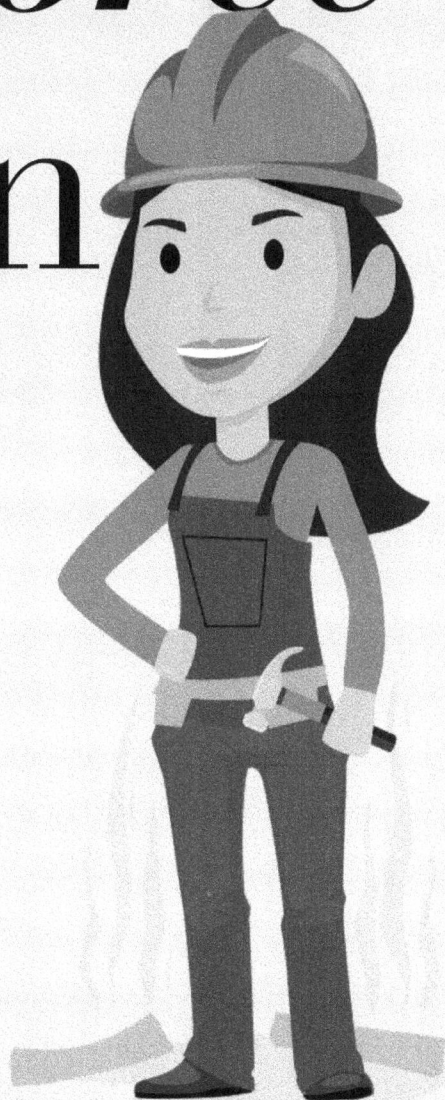

REINFORCE!

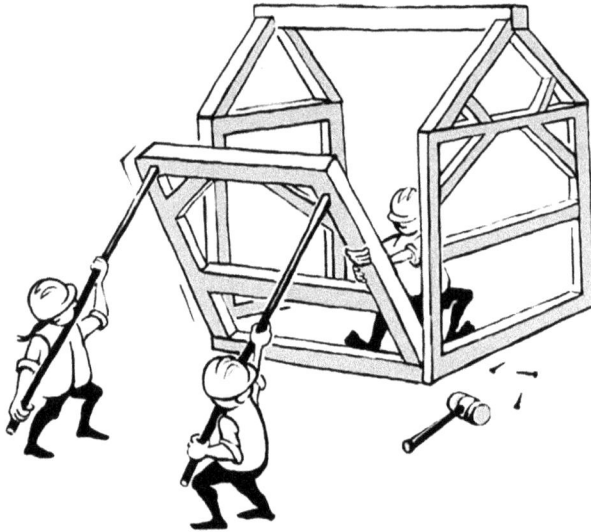

Q: *What* is being reinforced?

A: **Garbage-out transport systems for efficient elimination and cleanup**

Q: *How* will garbage-out transport systems be reinforced?

A: **By optimizing natural elimination processes**

➤ Go to the book for more: *Fix the Fire Damage*, pages 441 – 449

➤ Listen to the podcast: *Conversations About Everyday Pain*, Season 2, Episodes 40 - 42

NEXT STEPS:

1. Keep up with all your efforts for Body Chemistry Release and Retrain

2. Focus on getting the garbage out through all four exits:
   Colon • Bladder • Skin • Lungs

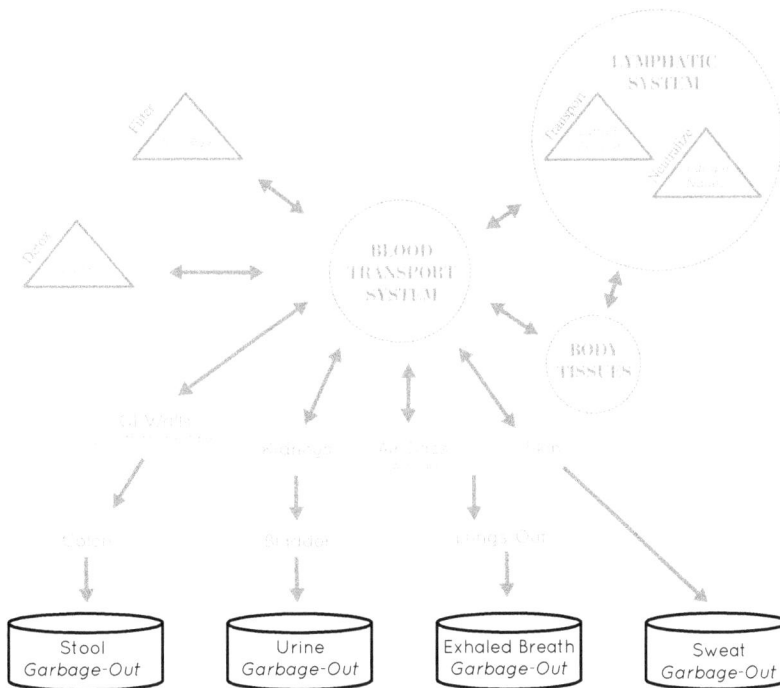

| Stool | Urine | Exhaled Breath | Sweat |
| Garbage-Out | Garbage-Out | Garbage-Out | Garbage-Out |

Get the Garbage Out!

Pick one or all four exits to focus on for 5-7 days while trying a few suggested strategies.

MY
ONE WEEK
BOWEL
JOURNAL

TODAY'S DATE: _____

 # OF BOWEL MOVEMENTS TODAY:_____

CONSISTENCY OF STOOL:
(circle one)

loose/unformed   soft/formed   hard & round

thin & long/formed

Other: _____

DIFFICULTY LEVEL:
(mark with an X)

TOOK A LONG TIME   SPEEDY EVACUATION

Notes:
Write about today's food, sleep, stress and/or your elimination schedule:

_____

_____

_____

_____

_____

MY ONE WEEK BOWEL JOURNAL

TODAY'S DATE: _____

 # OF BOWEL MOVEMENTS TODAY: _____

CONSISTENCY OF STOOL:
(circle one)

loose/unformed   soft/formed   hard & round

thin & long/formed

Other: _____

DIFFICULTY LEVEL:
(mark with an X)

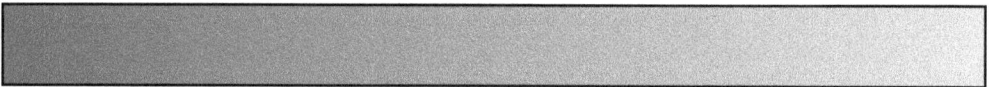

TOOK A LONG TIME   SPEEDY EVACUATION

Notes:
Write about today's food, sleep, stress and/or your elimination schedule:

_____

_____

_____

_____

_____

TODAY'S DATE: _____

 # OF BOWEL MOVEMENTS TODAY:_____

CONSISTENCY OF STOOL:
(circle one)

loose/unformed   soft/formed   hard & round

thin & long/formed

Other: _____

DIFFICULTY LEVEL:
(mark with an X)

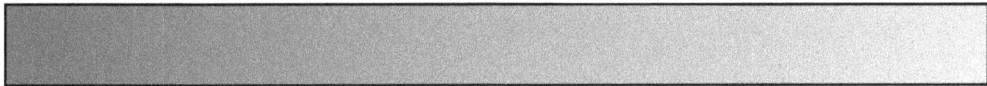

TOOK A LONG TIME   SPEEDY EVACUATION

Notes:
Write about today's food, sleep, stress and/or your elimination schedule:

_____

_____

_____

_____

_____

TODAY'S DATE: _____

 # OF BOWEL MOVEMENTS TODAY:_____

CONSISTENCY OF STOOL:
(circle one)

loose/unformed   soft/formed   hard & round

thin & long/formed

Other: _____

DIFFICULTY LEVEL:
(mark with an X)

TOOK A LONG TIME   SPEEDY EVACUATION

Notes:
Write about today's food, sleep, stress and/or your elimination schedule:

_____

_____

_____

_____

_____

TODAY'S DATE: _____

 # OF BOWEL MOVEMENTS TODAY: _____

CONSISTENCY OF STOOL:
(circle one)

> loose/unformed   soft/formed   hard & round
>
> thin & long/formed

Other: _____

DIFFICULTY LEVEL:
(mark with an X)

TOOK A LONG TIME   SPEEDY EVACUATION

Notes:
Write about today's food, sleep, stress and/or your elimination schedule:

_____

_____

_____

_____

_____

TODAY'S DATE: _____

OF BOWEL MOVEMENTS TODAY:_____

CONSISTENCY OF STOOL:
(circle one)

loose/unformed   soft/formed   hard & round

thin & long/formed

Other: _____

DIFFICULTY LEVEL:
(mark with an X)

TOOK A LONG TIME   SPEEDY EVACUATION

Notes:
Write about today's food, sleep, stress and/or your elimination schedule:

_____

_____

_____

_____

_____

TODAY'S DATE: _____

 # OF BOWEL MOVEMENTS TODAY: _____

CONSISTENCY OF STOOL:
(circle one)

loose/unformed   soft/formed   hard & round

thin & long/formed

Other: _____

DIFFICULTY LEVEL:
(mark with an X)

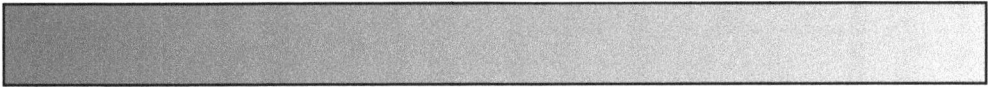

TOOK A LONG TIME   SPEEDY EVACUATION

Notes:
Write about today's food, sleep, stress and/or your elimination schedule:

_____

_____

_____

_____

_____

MY
ONE WEEK
BLADDER
JOURNAL

TODAY'S DATE: _____

 # OF PEE BREAKS: _____

AVERAGE LENGTH OF BLADDER EMPTYING:
(for a count of...)

Less than 5   Between 5 -10   Greater than 10

COLOR:
(circle one)

Clear   Pale Yellow   Bright Yellow   Dark Yellow   Brownish

Other: _____

Notes:
Write about today's beverages (what kind/how many) times you had to suppress the need to empty your bladder etc.

_____

_____

_____

_____

_____

_____

MY ONE WEEK BLADDER JOURNAL

TODAY'S DATE: _____

OF PEE BREAKS: _____

AVERAGE LENGTH OF BLADDER EMPTYING:
(for a count of...)

Less than 5   Between 5 -10   Greater than 10

COLOR:
(circle one)

Clear   Pale Yellow   Bright Yellow   Dark Yellow   Brownish

Other: _____

Notes:
Write about today's beverages (what kind/how many) times you had to suppress the need to empty your bladder etc.

_____

_____

_____

_____

_____

_____

TODAY'S DATE: _____

 # OF PEE BREAKS: _____

AVERAGE LENGTH OF BLADDER EMPTYING:
(for a count of...)

Less than 5   Between 5 -10   Greater than 10

COLOR:
(circle one)

Clear   Pale Yellow   Bright Yellow   Dark Yellow   Brownish

Other: _____

Notes:
Write about today's beverages (what kind/how many) times you had to suppress the need to empty your bladder etc.

_____

_____

_____

_____

_____

_____

TODAY'S DATE: _____

 # OF PEE BREAKS: _____

AVERAGE LENGTH OF BLADDER EMPTYING:
(for a count of...)

Less than 5   Between 5 -10   Greater than 10

COLOR:
(circle one)

Clear   Pale Yellow   Bright Yellow   Dark Yellow   Brownish

Other: _____

Notes:
Write about today's beverages (what kind/how many) times you had to suppress the need to empty your bladder etc.

_____

_____

_____

_____

_____

TODAY'S DATE: _____

 # OF PEE BREAKS: _____

AVERAGE LENGTH OF BLADDER EMPTYING:
(for a count of...)

Less than 5   Between 5 -10   Greater than 10

COLOR:
(circle one)

Clear   Pale Yellow   Bright Yellow   Dark Yellow   Brownish

Other: _____

Notes:
Write about today's beverages (what kind/how many) times you had to suppress the need to empty your bladder etc.

_____

_____

_____

_____

_____

_____

TODAY'S DATE: _____

 # OF PEE BREAKS: _____

AVERAGE LENGTH OF BLADDER EMPTYING:
(for a count of...)

Less than 5   Between 5 -10   Greater than 10

COLOR:
(circle one)

Clear   Pale Yellow   Bright Yellow   Dark Yellow   Brownish

Other: _____

Notes:
Write about today's beverages (what kind/how many) times you had to suppress the need to empty your bladder etc.

_____

_____

_____

_____

_____

_____

TODAY'S DATE: _____

 # OF PEE BREAKS: _____

AVERAGE LENGTH OF BLADDER EMPTYING:
(for a count of...)

      Less than 5   Between 5 -10   Greater than 10

COLOR:
(circle one)

  Clear   Pale Yellow   Bright Yellow   Dark Yellow   Brownish

Other: _____

Notes:
Write about today's beverages (what kind/how many) times you had to suppress the need to empty your bladder etc.

_____

_____

_____

_____

_____

_____

SEVEN DAYS OF SWEATING AND BREATHING

TODAY'S DATE: _____

What did I do to sweat or breathe mindfully today?
(Any kind of movement that creates heat counts. You don't have to feel sweaty.)

_____

_____

_____

_____

_____

_____

_____

_____

_____

_____

_____

Try setting an alarm 2-3 times a day to remind yourself to look up from your work and fill your belly with breath. Let your shoulders rise. Fill your upper back with air.

TODAY'S DATE: _____

What did I do to sweat or breathe mindfully today?

(Any kind of movement that creates heat counts. You don't have to feel sweaty.)

_____

_____

_____

_____

_____

_____

_____

_____

_____

_____

_____

Try setting an alarm 2-3 times a day to stand up or look up and into the distance. Squeeze your buttocks and release. Bang out 5-10 countertop push-ups on your desk or the kitchen counter.

TODAY'S DATE: _____

What did I do to sweat or breathe mindfully today?
(Any kind of movement that creates heat counts. You don't have to feel sweaty.)

_____

_____

_____

_____

_____

_____

_____

_____

_____

_____

_____

Did you manage to take yourself to the gym or did you ride your bike to work today, or did you take a walk around the block after dinner? Either way, well done! Celebrate!

TODAY'S DATE: _____

What did I do to sweat or breathe mindfully today?
(Any kind of movement that creates heat counts. You don't have to feel sweaty.)

_____

_____

_____

_____

_____

_____

_____

_____

_____

_____

_____

Try setting an alarm 2-3 times a day to stand up or look up and into the distance. Squeeze your buttocks and release. Bang out 5-10 countertop push-ups on your desk or the kitchen counter.

TODAY'S DATE: _____

What did I do to sweat or breathe mindfully today?
(Any kind of movement that creates heat counts. You don't have to feel sweaty.)

_____

_____

_____

_____

_____

_____

_____

_____

_____

_____

_____

Did you manage to take yourself to the gym or did you ride your bike to work today, or did you take a walk around the block after dinner? Either way, well done! Celebrate!

TODAY'S DATE: _____

What did I do to sweat or breathe mindfully today?
(Any kind of movement that creates heat counts. You don't have to feel sweaty.)

_____

_____

_____

_____

_____

_____

_____

_____

_____

_____

_____

Try setting an alarm 2-3 times a day to stand up or look up and into the distance. Squeeze your buttocks and release. Bang out 5-10 countertop push-ups on your desk or the kitchen counter.

TODAY'S DATE: _____

What did I do to sweat or breathe mindfully today?
(Any kind of movement that creates heat counts. You don't have to feel sweaty.)

_____

_____

_____

_____

_____

_____

_____

_____

_____

_____

_____

_____

Did you manage to take yourself to the gym or did you ride your bike to work today, or did you take a walk around the block after dinner? Either way, well done! Celebrate!

My Everyday Pain Story

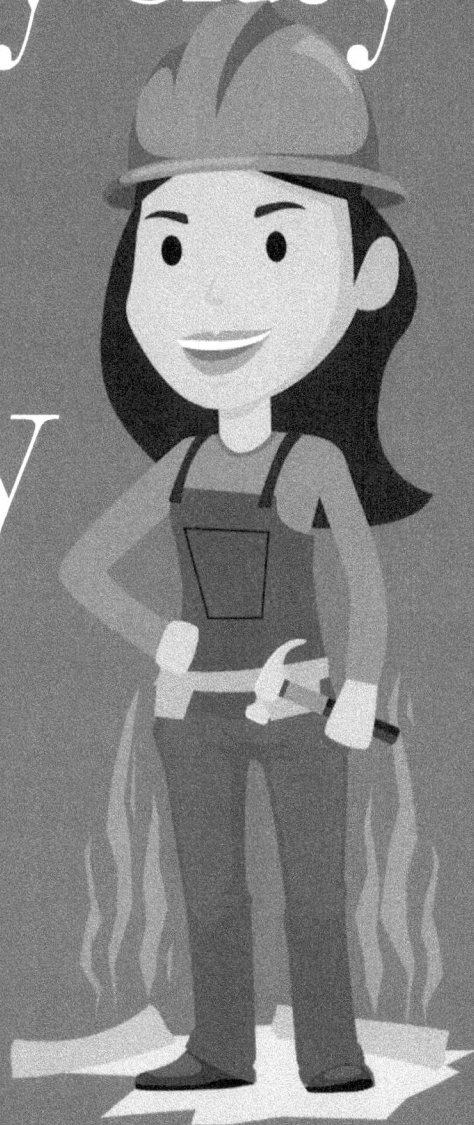

My Everyday Pain Story

When I have less pain, I look forward to...
doing/feeling/being:

_____

_____

_____

_____

_____

_____

_____

_____

_____

_____

_____

My Everyday Pain Story

When I am less inflamed, I look forward to...
doing/feeling/being:

_____

_____

_____

_____

_____

_____

_____

_____

_____

_____

_____

My Everyday Pain Story

My first or most memorable pain
experience or injury as a child

_____

_____

_____

_____

_____

_____

_____

_____

_____

_____

_____

What part of me was hurt?

How did it happen?

Who was there with me or was I alone?

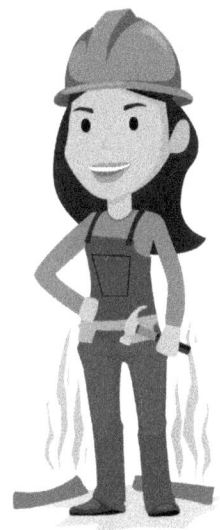

My Everyday Pain Story

If there was a parent, guardian, friend or teacher nearby, how did they react to my injury?

If I was alone at the time, how did I feel about that?

Were any of these feelings present: shame, blame, anger, fear, embarrassment, humor, achievement?

Notes:

_____

_____

_____

_____

_____

_____

_____

_____

_____

_____

_____

_____

_____

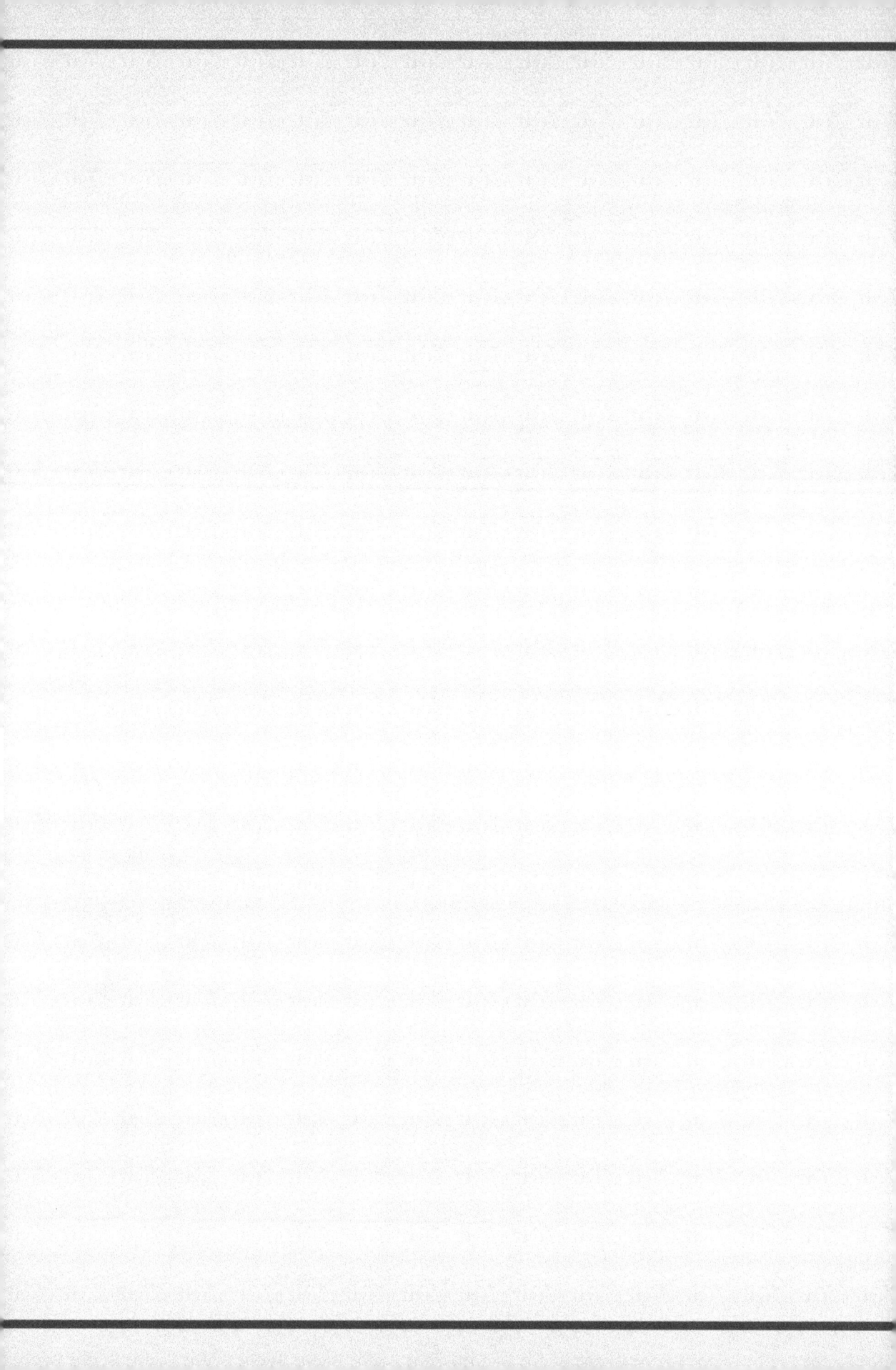

What
the
Pros
Say

A Question and Answer
Session with the Pros

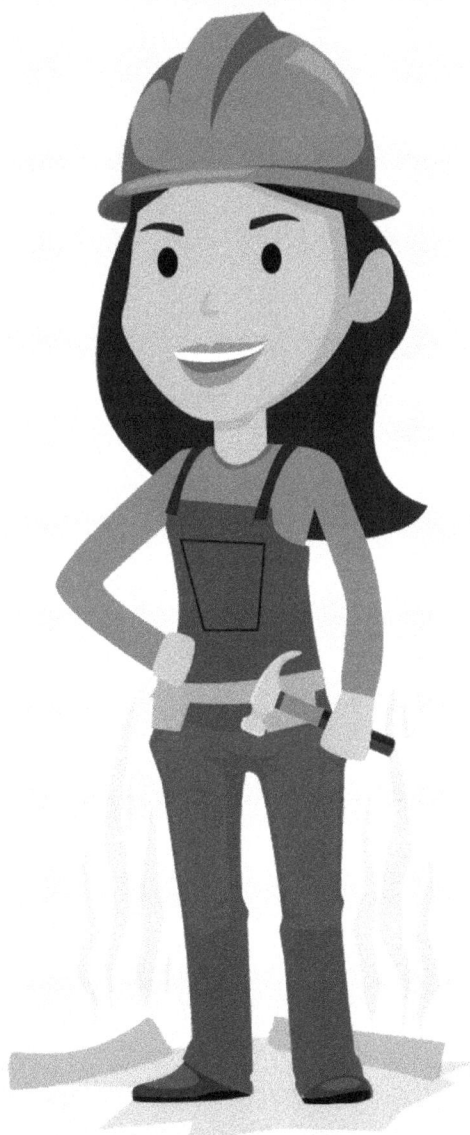

WHAT THE PROS SAY

WHAT FOLLOWS NEXT IS A COLLECTION of perspectives from a small sampling of providers in different health disciplines. These four voices are practitioners local to Seattle, Washington, who kindly responded to my request for contributions to this book series. I'm sharing the insights of these professionals in three different disciplines (naturopathic, allopathic functional medicine, and Eastern medicine) about their individual approaches to treating pain, specifically from the point of view taken when working directly or indirectly with body chemistry through either nutrients, food, herbs, or pharmaceutical medication. I urge you to use some of the questions addressed here as a jumping off point as you consider your next phase in the pain repair process, which may include any one of these areas in healthcare to help you explore your unique body chemistry needs.

Please note that none of this is an endorsement for or against a specific modality or method. Rather, this section will primarily show you a small sampling of existing care options. At the end of this chapter, you'll see my personal take on what the bottom line might be. While each interview was unique, there are a few common threads that you might also detect as you read through them.

MEET THE PROS

Christy Lee-Engel, ND, LAc

www.lifecultivatinglife.com

Licensed as a naturopathic physician since 1992
and as an acupuncturist since 1995, acupuncture
has become her primary therapeutic mode. Dr.
Lee-Engel also offers careful listening and gentle
guidance, support, and recommendations as her
patients explore how to develop and sustain healthier lifestyle habits.

Adjunct faculty member at Bastyr University (1994 to 2019). Assistant
Dean in the School of Naturopathic Medicine (2002 to 2004). Founding
Director of the Bastyr University Center for Mind, Body, Spirit, and Nature
(2009-2016).

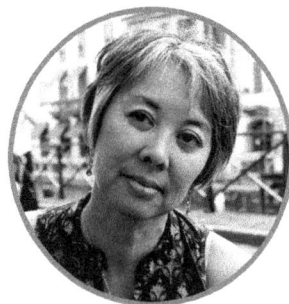

Steven M. Hall, MD

www.stevenmhallmd.com

Steven M. Hall, MD, began his medical career in
1985 as a residency trained and board-certified
Family Practitioner. He is the author of *The Seven
Tools of Healing*. Since 1991, Dr. Hall has been an
adjunct professor and clinical preceptor of Natu-
ropathic Medicine for Bastyr University. For many years, he also has been

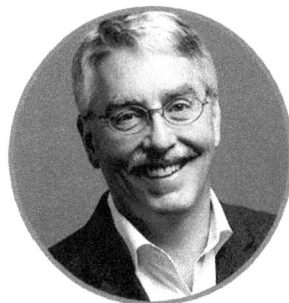

teaching comprehensive craniosacral therapy training and varied specific wellness classes in other settings.

His practice has been strongly influenced by his search for the answers to two questions: "What is 'healing'?" and "How can I best help you with yours?" His search quickly took him beyond the borders of conventional medicine, and he has explored many of the world's leading healing traditions. He excels at taking seemingly disparate and conflicting ideas, finding common ground, and integrating them.

He has developed and currently practices a form of medicine that successfully integrates the best from conventional and many forms of alternative medicine into one seamless medicine.

Paige Barnes, LAc

www.peonymedicine.com

Paige Barnes is an East Asian Medicine Practitioner, dance artist, and founder of Peony. Her practice focuses on preventative care, pain management, mental health, and rehabilitation. She believes acupuncture and herbal medicine return us to listening to and caring for ourselves, each other, and the natural world.

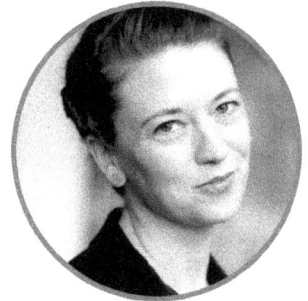

Paige applies over 20 years of experience as a dance artist and Gyrotonic instructor to her clinical viewpoint. Dance and Gyrotonic cultivate how to listen, feel, and see our body's poetry—its imagination and history, and its story. East Asian Medicine philosophy cultivates an awareness of how our health is in relationship to the natural world. Integrating and applying the worldview of these disciplines creates a compassionate space for self-discovery, self-acceptance, and self-restoration.

Paige holds an MS in East Asian Medicine from Bastyr University, 2016, and a BA in Dance from the University of Washington, 1999. She continues her Chinese Medicine education through Neijing Nature-Based

Medicine with Dr. Edward Neal, recently completing the Level 1 program in 2021.

Melinda Bower, ND

www.drmelindabower.com

Dr. Melinda Bower is a naturopathic and functional medicine doctor in Seattle and Port Townsend, Washington. With advanced training in women's health, autoimmune disorders, cognitive impairment, and personalized medicine, Dr. Bower specializes in identifying hormone imbalances, nutrient deficiencies, food reactions, environmental triggers, and the prevention of chronic disease overall.

This approach involves finding and treating the source of the problem, symptoms, or disease—rather than just treating the symptoms—in order to create sustained healing.

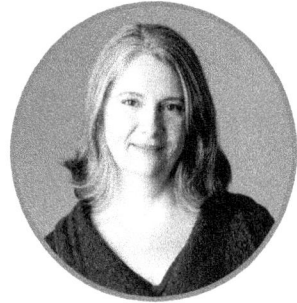

ASK THE PROS

Ask the Pros

How would you describe your role to someone seeking help for chronic recurring aches and pains?

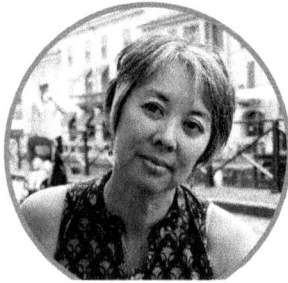

I help people to feel more at ease and to experience less pain and stressful effects in their lives, using primarily acupuncture and lifestyle counseling combined with herbal, nutritional, homeopathic medicines, and a wide range of resources and referrals.

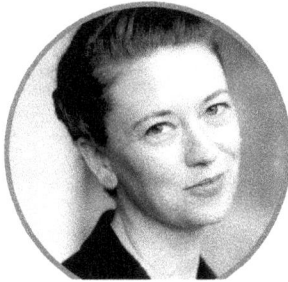

Christy Lee-Engel, ND, LAc

I aim to create a comfortable and safe environment for people to be heard. I accept the person's narrative about their pain as reality because their perception is legitimate, and it's their personal truth. I offer an approach to shift the pain pattern from a Chinese medicine perspective that supports the emotional and energetic body. I believe it is important for the patient to accept

Paige Barnes, LAc

the possibility of pain relief from acupuncture before engaging in the practice. I ask the patient to subjectively measure their pain, and I record that impression. If the said pain decreases through the treatments, I point this out during our work together to give reassurance in their body's ability to heal itself. In addition, I emphasize the process of healing as opposed to fixing, which is a dynamic process that takes time, patience, gentleness, and compassion with oneself.

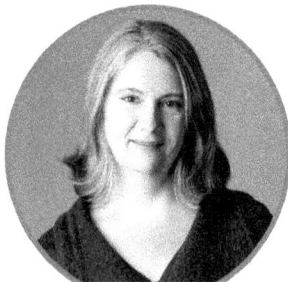

I mostly gather information and refer to the appropriate person who I think can best help them with that symptom.

Melinda Bower, ND

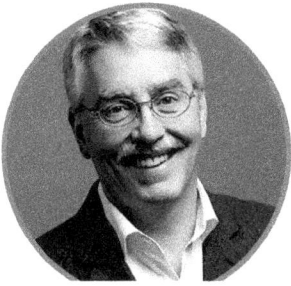

Steven M. Hall, M.D.

I use functional and integrative medical concepts, diagnostics, and treatments to find and treat the root causes of your symptoms, including your pain.

Your body/mind/energy has much more healing and regenerative power than our culture gives it credit for. I help you find and stop the forces in your life that cause your system to degenerate, including self-sabotage, poor diet, stress, poor quality sleep, etc., While we work to nurture and support the forces that cause your system to regenerate, including creating the underlying beliefs and motivations you need to sustain a good diet, appropriate exercise, restful sleep, personal empowerment, healthy relationships, etc.

I also employ advanced craniosacral therapy as a hands-on way to help you release fascial restrictions, muscle tension patterns, improve alignment, access your body memory, uncover and release limiting beliefs, direct your stem cells to areas that need repair, access your own deep knowing, and much more.

I also have years of experience helping people successfully wean off addictive medications once the above approach makes them unnecessary.

Ask the Pros

How do you feel about working with patients who are concurrently also receiving other care (acupuncture, massage, chiropractic, physical therapy, psychotherapy, other)? Do you and it affects outcomes positively or negatively?

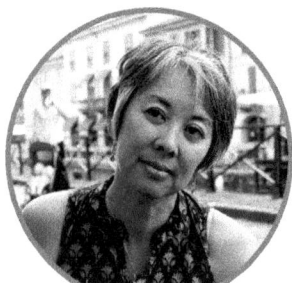

Christy Lee-Engel, ND, LAc

I almost always work with patients as part of their healthcare team, whether or not I am in direct touch with their other practitioners. Knowing what kind of other therapies they are receiving helps me to tailor my treatments in terms of timing, intensity, areas worked on in a given week. I often see patients benefiting from combinations of care, either adding acupuncture to what wasn't quite working before, or adding another type of therapy to acupuncture and reaching new levels of positive results!

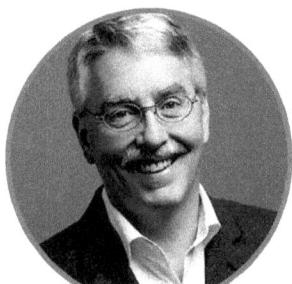

Steven M. Hall, M.D.

Most of my patients already utilize one or more additional forms of care, and if they don't, I often refer where and when it is appropriate. Most chronically pained people do better with the support of a carefully selected team of committed professionals.

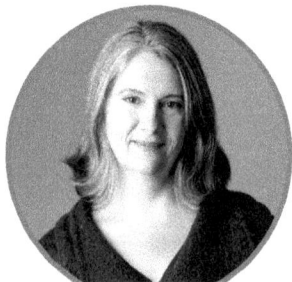

Melinda Bower, ND

I prefer my patients to have a care team that includes acupuncture, massage, chiropractic, physical therapy, and counseling if needed. I always find a good team approach is super helpful.

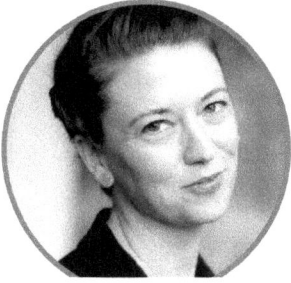

Paige Barnes, LAc

I enjoy working with someone who is also working with other practitioners. I enjoy it even more if I know the practitioners and their style and have the ability to communicate and learn from their treatments and approaches. If a person is actively engaged in their healing process, I believe a team of practitioners who are coming from different perspectives is beneficial.

Depending on the case, I like the combination of acupuncture, naturopathy, physical medicine (chiropractor, physical therapy), psychotherapy, and a primary care physician. I think physical medicine, psychotherapy, and acupuncture are important types of care to have regularly in one's life for management and prevention while an ND and MD are less frequent check-ins. I think as long as the collective practitioners trust each other's insight and care, the outcome is favorable.

Ask the Pros

Do you counsel patients/clients about how to coordinate integrative care with other professionals? If so, what are your common recommendations?

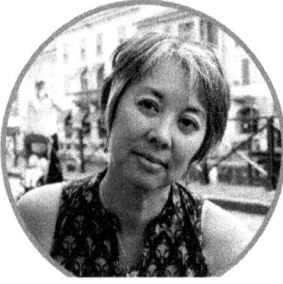

Yes, but in my experience, it all depends on the patient (what their situation is, how sensitive they are), and I don't have any "one-size-fits-all" recommendation. I have seen massage and acupuncture work well together on the same day or spaced a week or two apart, and the same for chiropractic care or physical therapy plus acupuncture. Patients will oftentimes figure out the best schedule for themselves.

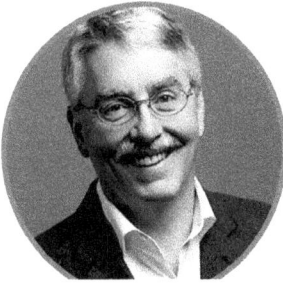

Christy Lee-Engel, ND, LAc

To get the best outcome and reduce the risk of wasting time, money, and resources, I think a person's support team should be assembled with the guidance of a well-trained integrative medical professional who knows the patient well and is familiar with all the other modalities, what they have to offer, who in the community is good at them, how to time them with the patient's current state and progress and such.

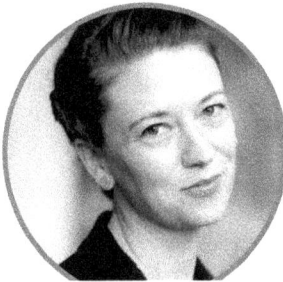

Steven M. Hall, M.D.

Yes. I have familiarity with coordinating integrative care between acupuncture and naturopathy as well as acupuncture and chiropractic care. I commonly advise naturopathic care for blood work to be taken and reviewed, an overview of desired health outcomes, a review of current supplements and pharmaceuticals, digestive function, and hormone health. I also enjoy receiving feedback from providers like a chiropractor on a patient's process while receiving acupuncture care. Structural manipulation is synergistic with energetic medicine.

Paige Barnes, LAc

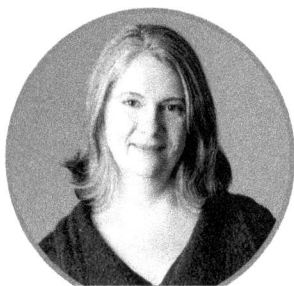

Melinda Bower, ND

Yes, I also send referrals to support this and am happy to consult with other practitioners.

Ask the Pros

Do you make lifestyle recommendations? If so, are there one or two that you recommend more often than others and why?

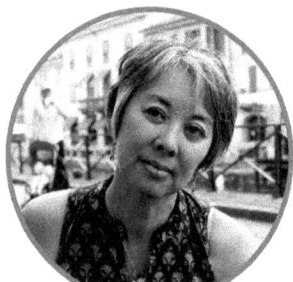

Yes, for almost everyone I work with. Often, they (recommendations) will be around the related topics of sleep/ rest and activity/exercise. I often talk with patients about "sleep hygiene" and explore what would help them sleep better (dark room, cool temperature, ways of winding down, and decreasing screen exposure before bed, timing

Christy Lee-Engel, ND, LAc

of meals, etc.) and sleep longer. Acupuncture can be helpful for sleep disturbances, too, as well as helping people realign their circadian rhythms. As far as movement and exercise, I often talk with patients about ways of incorporating more movement into their day that doesn't necessarily depend on going to a gym, including the use of fitness trackers or timers on their computers, etc. Also stretching exercises that can be easily done at work. For people with injuries or chronic pain, I also often recommend contrast hydrotherapy, to increase circulation, calm the nervous system, and thereby decrease discomfort and inflammation.

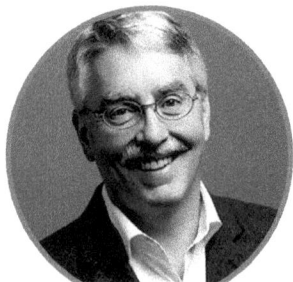

A person's lifestyle is the result of their world view. To make lasting, meaningful changes in lifestyle, the patient needs to first make lasting, meaningful changes in their world view. A person's world view is composed of all of the conclusions they've drawn, all the beliefs that they hold. Most worldview determining beliefs are held in

Steven M. Hall, M.D.

the unconscious mind. The person doesn't necessarily know they are there; they just see their results as what they think is reality. To make lifestyle changes, a person needs a way to go into their unconscious mind, find the limiting beliefs, bring them into the light of the conscious mind, align the belief with higher truth, then put the new belief back into the unconscious mind. Changes then just make sense and do not create resistance, feelings of deprivation, or risk going back to their old ways. I have found a way to do all this with my patients. What changes they make to their lifestyle are informed by their higher knowing.

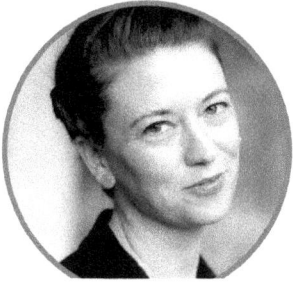

Paige Barnes, LAc

Yes. Walks; journaling; Epsom salt baths; recipes: sugar free treats, bone broth, and nutritious smoothies; nutrition from a TCM (Traditional Chinese Medicine) perspective like oysters to support kidney function and eating in alignment with the season; going to sleep by 11pm; a nighttime-before-bed routine; stretches to open low back and hips; cook books; Gyrotonic exercise system... Mostly, I think people need more gentle and nutritious activities and foods in their life. I encourage anything that can support those choices.

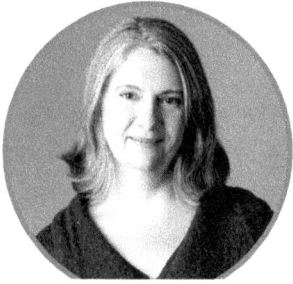

Melinda Bower, ND

Yes, mostly in relation to nutrition, sleep, exercise, stress management, and self-care.

Ask the Pros

Are there any other common "homework" tasks (behavior modification) that you require of your patients/clients while under your care?

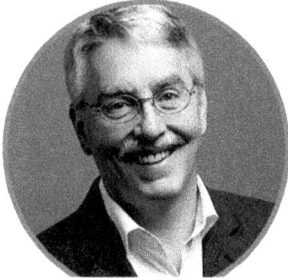

Behavior modification is working on the surface, which is way too superficial to get to the real roots of problems. I do ask my patients to practice paying attention to their bodies, minds, feelings, actions, relationships, and other aspects of their life. I then show them how to use all that information to get to know themselves better and make more heart-centered choices for themselves.

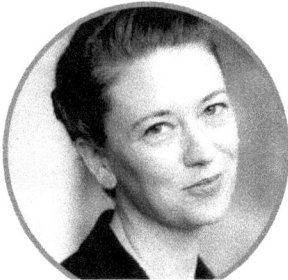

Steven M. Hall, M.D.

Requiring someone to do a task is difficult. If I think their choices are placing their body and health in a dangerous place, then I will require a shift or seeing a specialist who can more appropriately address an emergency condition. Otherwise, I suggest and explain a recommendation and why it would be beneficial. The patient needs to be excited about this idea in order for it to integrate into their life.

Paige Barnes, LAc

If there is not motivation to make a shift in a pain pattern, I will not recommend or force anything. It is important for the patient to ask, to inquire, and to be involved in their health before I make suggestions. Often to create a shift in pain, especially if chronic, involves significant lifestyle changes. This requires a slow, step by step process and often a paradigm shift on how to be in the world. If attempted all at once, it is rejected.

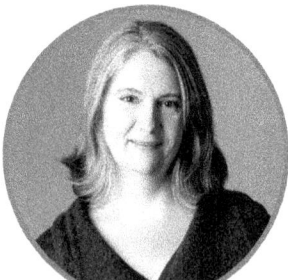

I focus on lifestyle pieces that are missing and supporting those things. I discuss all of the items [nutrition, sleep, exercise, stress management, and self-care] at least once with every patient.

Melinda Bower, ND

Has there ever been a situation where you would turn someone away or redirect them to a different therapy/modality? If so, please explain the circumstances.

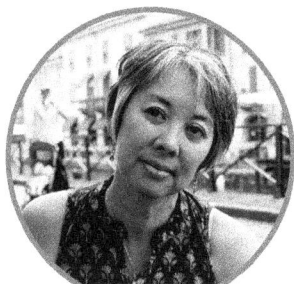

I often suggest to folks with hip or neck pain to also seek chiropractic care as, in my experience, it can be the best approach (and for some people the combination of chiropractic and acupuncture is the best).

Christy Lee-Engel, ND, LAc

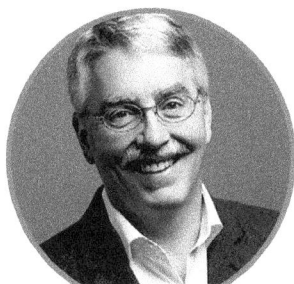

In thirty-three years of practice, I have only discharged four patients. One kept no-showing her appointments (at least eight), and I finally had to tell her that I couldn't care for her if she didn't come in. The other three were lying to me to get controlled substances and were not interested in or willing to do the work to heal themselves. I do refer people to other practitioners if they need or could benefit from something I don't offer.

Steven M. Hall, M.D.

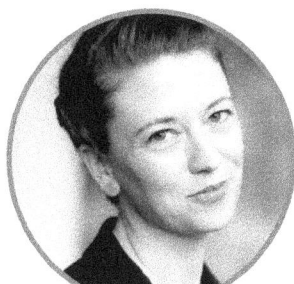

Not yet! I think people naturally self-select their treatment process. However, if after five treatments, I do not see any shift and/or if I notice an apathetic and resistant behavior to the care, I would recommend a different modality.

Paige Barnes, LAc

Ask the Pros

Is there a particular pain condition or variety of pain that you enjoy working with/have good success with? If so, please elaborate.

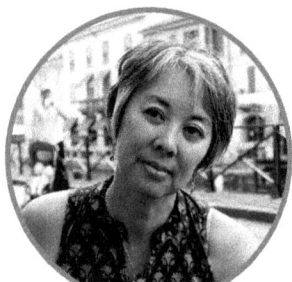

Christy Lee-Engel, ND, LAc

I've seen especially good results with knee pain and shoulder pain and sometimes with sciatica. I also like working with people who have headaches of various kinds to try to figure out what the causative factors are.

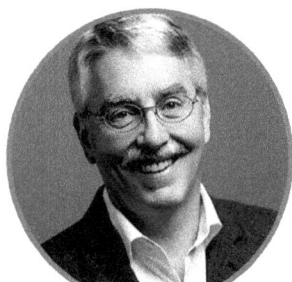

Steven M. Hall, M.D.

I've had good success with headaches (in fact, I believe no one needs to live with headaches; there is almost always a way to find and resolve the cause). I also work extensively with fibromyalgia and have an e-book on it available on Amazon. I've also had good results with complex regional pain syndromes and reflex sympathetic dystrophy. I have a special interest in low back pain and neck pain. So, I guess, not really. I don't specialize in any organ system or set of conditions; I specialize more in a way of problem-solving that can be applied to just about any condition.

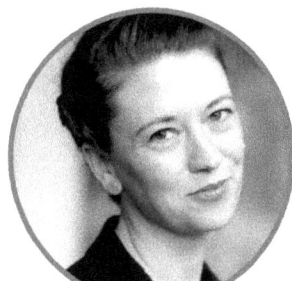

Paige Barnes, LAc

This is hard to answer quickly. I enjoy helping to alleviate all types of pain: emotional and physical. It has been rewarding for me to work with professional dancers, being a part of their care team when recovering from a serious injury and to see them perform again. I find it rewarding to assist someone who is committed to their health, taking responsibility for it, in order to engage in life activities that are meaningful for them.

Do you feel that your area of expertise (in regard to pain) relates in some way directly or indirectly to patients' experience of inflammation? If so, how?

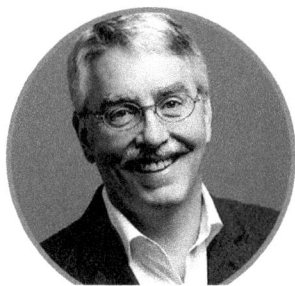

Steven M. Hall, M.D.

I always address inflammation, or being in a pro-inflammatory state, in all my patients. Some common roots involve leaky gut or some other cause of long-term activation of the immune system, of which there are several that I look for. Inflammation doesn't generally happen to someone in a vacuum; usually, we can find and treat the cause(s) of autoimmunity, allergy, and long-term activation of the mucosal-associated lymphoid tissue. If symptomatic treatment is needed, I've got years of experience with low-dose naltrexone, curcumin, Boswellia, contrast hydrotherapy, and other natural anti-inflammatories. NSAIDs are usually reserved for a last resort or patient preference.

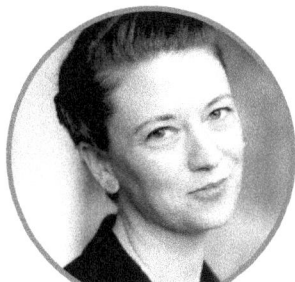

Paige Barnes, LAc

From a Chinese medicine perspective, the concept of inflammation is treated indirectly. When looking at a swollen area, I ask myself, "Is this hot or cold? Is this coming from a yin or yang deficiency? Is this coming from an excess of dampness? Does this relate to an organ's channel imbalance such as the spleen, liver, kidney, and/or heart channel system?"

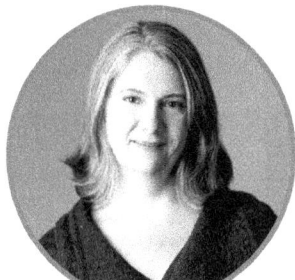

Melinda Bower, ND

I think most pain is from inflammation, and I do support that with lifestyle and sometimes anti-inflammatory herbs.

Ask the Pros

Are there common misconceptions about your profession or your work that you encounter with patients? If so, how would you like to see/hear that clarified?

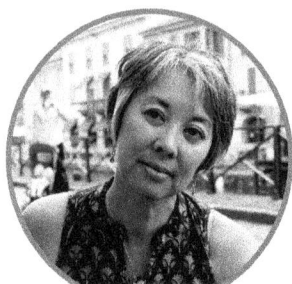

Christy Lee-Engel, ND, LAc

While acupuncture can certainly be considered an "invasive" therapy, the needles used are extremely fine and tiny compared to the needles used to give shots or draw blood! Acupuncture treatments are in general very relaxing—many patients fall asleep during treatment—no matter what the condition is that we are treating.

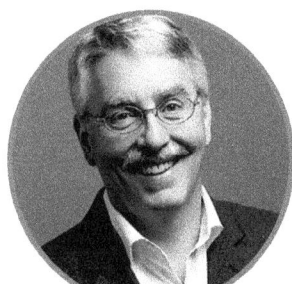

Steven M. Hall, M.D.

Many people think that craniosacral therapy just treats the head when, in reality, it is so versatile and powerful it could be its own system of medicine, as are homeopathy, chiropractic, and acupuncture.

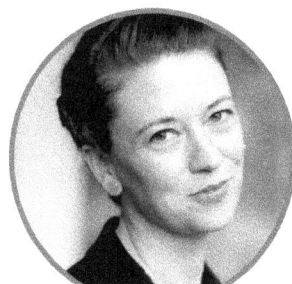

Paige Barnes, LAc

I am still learning about people's perceptions of acupuncture. I am fortunate to work in Seattle where, for the most part, there is an understanding and acceptance of Chinese medicine. Generally, the people who walk through my door believe in the healing capabilities of the medicine's philosophy. With this said, most people come in due to musculoskeletal pain. Chinese medicine can be utilized for internal medicine like gynecology, mental health, urogenital health, upper respiratory health, gastrointestinal health, pre- and post-operative care, fatigue, insomnia, migraines, stress, and in general it is effective at supporting the body's health while undergoing treatments for serious conditions such as cancer.

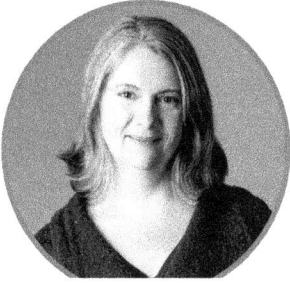

Melinda Bower, ND

Some people don't know that naturopathic physicians can be primary care providers or that we learn about many different modalities because not every naturopathic physician uses all of the modalities in practice, so it's complicated and can be confusing for everyday people.

The Take-Aways

➤ Ease, comfort, and safety are some of the common goals in treatment.

➤ Collaboration between providers and disciplines of care, whether intentional or incidental, is welcomed and encouraged.

➤ Lifestyle changes around sleep, stress management, movement, breathing, and nourishment are a must for success.

➤ Many of us providers take oaths to open our doors to anyone and everyone, but it's natural to develop special interests and strengths for certain types of clinical cases. It's a completely fair question for a patient to inquire about when interviewing a prospective healthcare provider.

➤ Impacting inflammation can happen through many different avenues, but there seems to be some consensus that doing so is directly and indirectly part of care when pain is at play.

➤ As a patient, it might be useful to set aside preconceived notions about certain disciplines of healthcare because no two practitioners deliver the same experience of human interaction. The therapeutic relationship can be as unique as each human being.

As you can see, there are a number of modalities that any single healthcare provider will use to address pain and the underlying contributing factors – some of which may have to do with inflammation and your body chemistry. Of course, if you've been navigating this book series, you know that it includes an entire section and separate workbook dedicated to the role that stress biology and emotions play when dealing with pain. So you also know that your body chemistry doesn't operate in a vacuum. At the end of the third companion manual, *Fix Your Stress Biology*, you'll see a new group of "pros" who share with you their perspectives on pain from a mental health and brain biology vantage point.

MAKE THE MOST OF
YOUR VISIT

Questions to ask when checking out new practitioners to aid with biochemical health:

1. How do you see your role in this process?

2. What are your expectations of me?

3. Is there a timeline with milestones to reach for?

4. How do you measure progress and when do I know it's time to move on?

5. How often do you see and work with clinical cases like mine?

A few things you should prepare to share with your practitioners:

1. Communicate your pain with as many specific, descriptive adjectives as possible.

2. Pay attention to the situations and time of day when you notice your pain the most.

3. Remember which of the Action Plan strategies provided relief.

4. Be honest about the things you might be consciously taking into your body-machine that you know are not ideal. You are human.

Food
Ideas
Lists

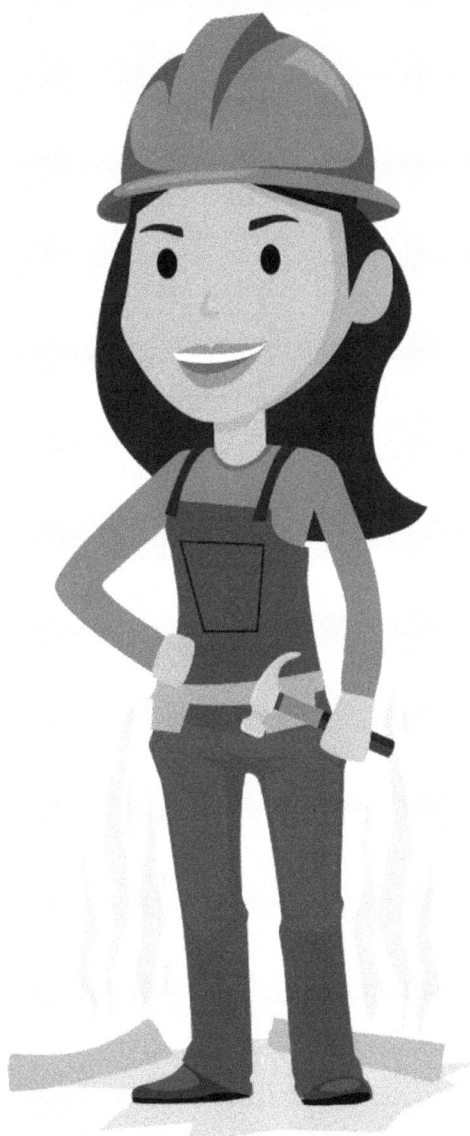

LOW GLYCEMIC INDEX FOOD IDEAS[1]

MOST VEGETABLES:

- [ ] Green peas
- [ ] Onions
- [ ] Lettuce
- [ ] Cabbage
- [ ] Leafy greens such as spinach, collards, kale, and beet
- [ ] Green beans
- [ ] Tomatoes
- [ ] Cucumbers
- [ ] Bok choy
- [ ] Artichokes
- [ ] Brussels sprouts
- [ ] Broccoli
- [ ] Cauliflower
- [ ] Celery
- [ ] Eggplant
- [ ] Peppers including bell peppers and jalapenos
- [ ] Zucchini
- [ ] Crookneck squash
- [ ] Snow peas
- [ ] Mushrooms

CERTAIN FRUITS:

- [ ] Apples
- [ ] Pears
- [ ] Plum
- [ ] Avocado
- [ ] Olives
- [ ] Dried apricots
- [ ] Unripe banana
- [ ] Peaches
- [ ] Strawberries
- [ ] Oranges
- [ ] Cherries
- [ ] Coconut
- [ ] Grapefruit
- [ ] Cranberries
- [ ] Blueberries

1. https://www.medicinenet.com/low-glycemic_foods_list_guide/article.htm

WHOLE OR MINIMALLY PROCESSED GRAINS:

- [ ] Barley
- [ ] Whole wheat
- [ ] Oat bran and rice bran cereals
- [ ] Whole-grain pasta
- [ ] Whole-grain pumpernickel bread
- [ ] Sourdough bread
- [ ] Wheat tortilla

DAIRY AND DAIRY SUBSTITUTE PRODUCTS

- [ ] Plain yogurt
- [ ] Cheese
- [ ] Cottage cheese
- [ ] Milk
- [ ] Soy milk and yogurt

MISCELLANEOUS

- [ ] Nuts and nut butter
- [ ] Seeds such as pumpkin, chia, sunflower, and flax seeds
- [ ] Poultry such as chicken and turkey
- [ ] Eggs and egg whites
- [ ] Fish and shellfish
- [ ] Meat such as beef and pork
- [ ] Oils such as extra virgin olive oil and canola oil
- [ ] Fats such as lard, shortening, and butter
- [ ] Mayonnaise

HIGH FIBER FOOD IDEAS

FRUITS

- [ ] Raspberries
- [ ] Pear
- [ ] Apple, with skin
- [ ] Banana
- [ ] Orange
- [ ] Strawberries

GRAINS

- [ ] Spaghetti, whole-wheat, cooked
- [ ] Barley, pearled, cooked
- [ ] Bran flakes
- [ ] Quinoa, cooked
- [ ] Oat bran muffins
- [ ] Oatmeal, instant, cooked
- [ ] Popcorn, air-popped
- [ ] Brown rice, cooked
- [ ] Bread, whole-wheat
- [ ] Bread, rye

VEGETABLES

- [ ] Green peas, boiled
- [ ] Broccoli, boiled
- [ ] Turnip greens, boiled
- [ ] Brussels sprouts, boiled
- [ ] Sweet corn, boiled
- [ ] Cauliflower, raw
- [ ] Carrot, raw

LEGUMES, NUTS AND SEEDS

- [ ] Split peas, boiled
- [ ] Lentils, boiled
- [ ] Black beans, boiled
- [ ] Cannellini, Navy, Great Norther beans, canned
- [ ] Chia seeds
- [ ] Almonds
- [ ] Pistachios
- [ ] Sunflower kernels

MINERAL RICH FOOD IDEAS

- [ ] Nuts and seeds
- [ ] Shellfish
- [ ] Cruciferous vegetables
- [ ] Organ meats
- [ ] Eggs
- [ ] Beans
- [ ] Cocoa
- [ ] Avocados
- [ ] Berries
- [ ] Yogurt
- [ ] Cheese
- [ ] Sardines
- [ ] Spirulina
- [ ] Ancient grains (amaranth, millet, quinoa)
- [ ] Starchy vegetables (sweet potatoes, butternut squash)
- [ ] Tropical fruits
- [ ] Leafy greens

ABOUT THE AUTHOR

YA-LING J. LIOU, DC, is a chiropractic physician who, after more than 30 years of clinical experience, continues to expand and share her intuitive body care techniques. All of her work takes into account the whole person, aiming not only to address the mechanical balance of the body, but also the chemical and emotional aspects that so often influence this balance.

Growing up with exposure to generations of Eastern as well as Western attitudes toward health has provided Dr. Liou with a unique perspective on health care. She began her formal education in the area of applied sciences in her hometown of Montreal, Quebec, before completing a degree program at New York Chiropractic College.

Dr. Liou now lives, works, and writes in Seattle. She taught anatomy, physiology and kinesiology at Seattle Massage School (currently Everest College and formerly Ashmead College) and later brought her multiple-systems perspective to the Naturopathic Physical Medicine Department at Bastyr University as an adjunct faculty member.

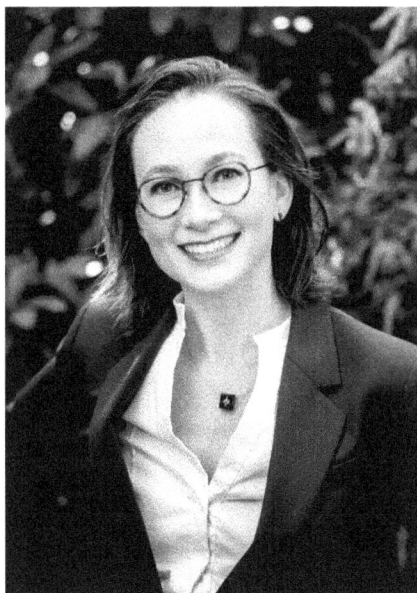

Want to learn more? Stay connected with the author by visitng www.ya-ling.com.

www.ingramcontent.com/pod-product-compliance
Lightning Source LLC
Chambersburg PA
CBHW051323020426
42333CB00032B/3461